Acknowledgment

I would like to give my gratitude to my mom for the delicious food, my husband Sabbah & my kids Omar, Mohannad, Nadine & Ashly, my brothers and sisters, and all of my family and friends who encouraged me to proceed with the book. Special thanks to Nadine Afiouni, Zeina Makhoul, John Archuleta, Martha Kern, Suzanne Cummins, Mariam Adra, Nabil Khoury and every single person who came to my home and had bread and butter with us. You are welcome anytime.

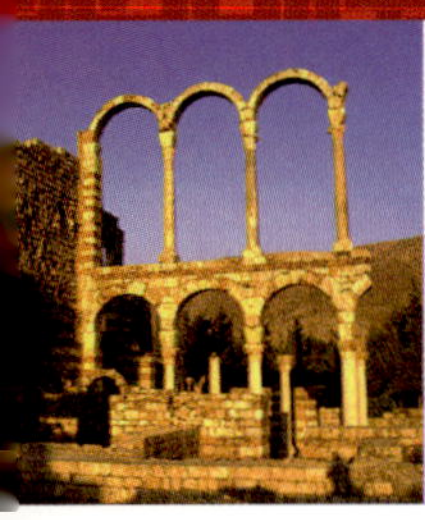
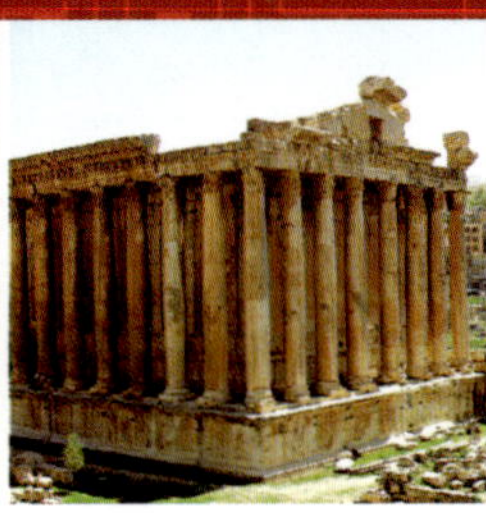
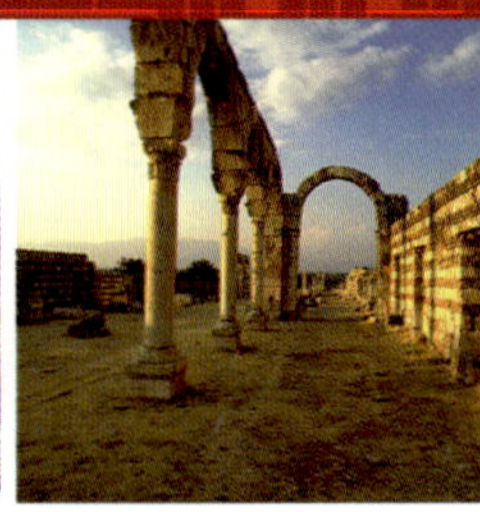
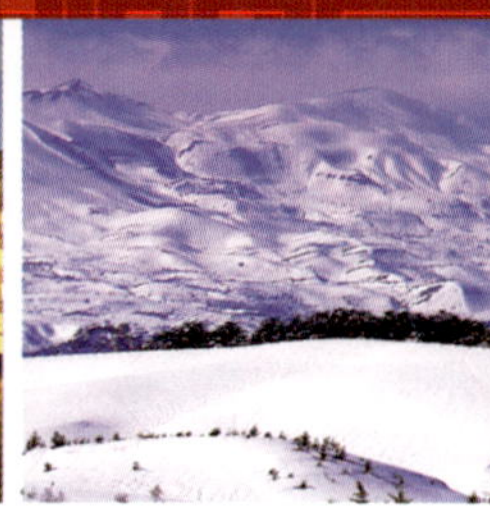
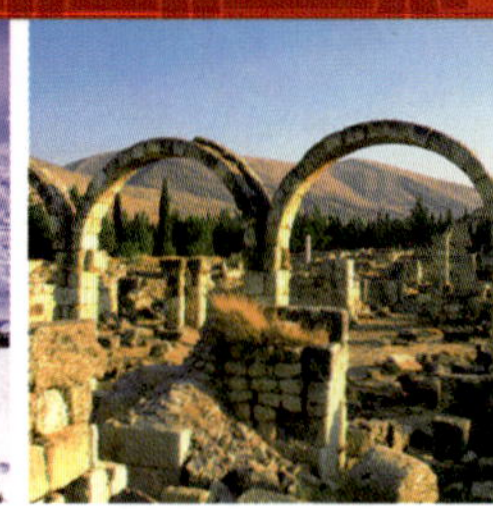
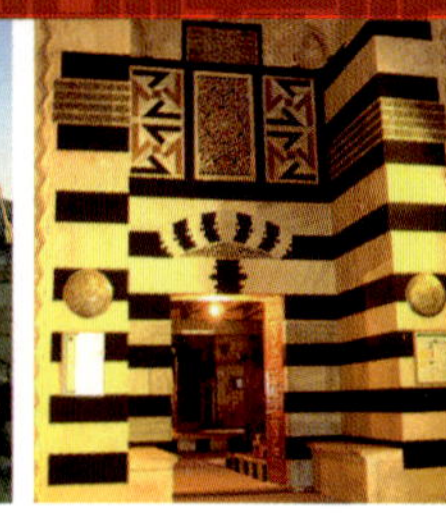

THE PURE TASTE OF LEBANON FROM SAFA'S KITCHEN

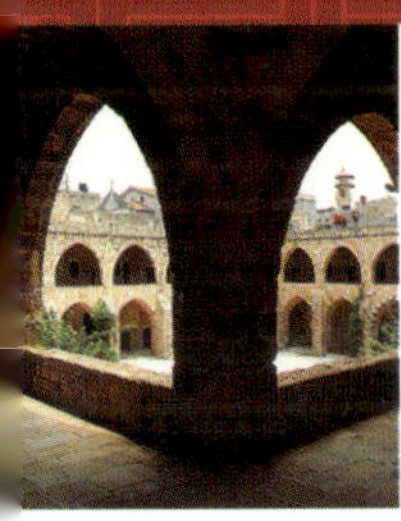
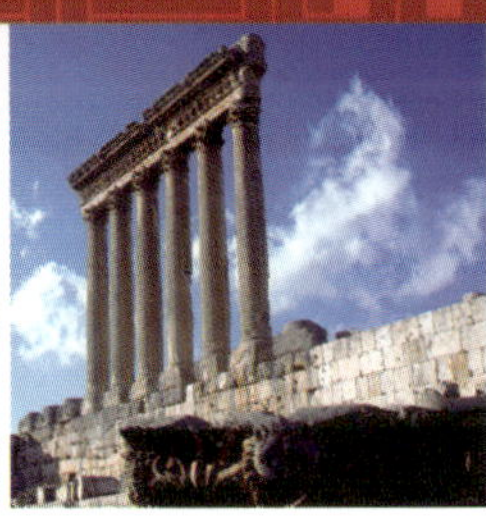
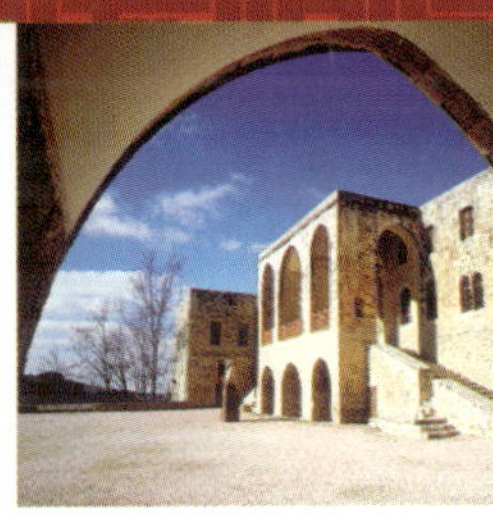
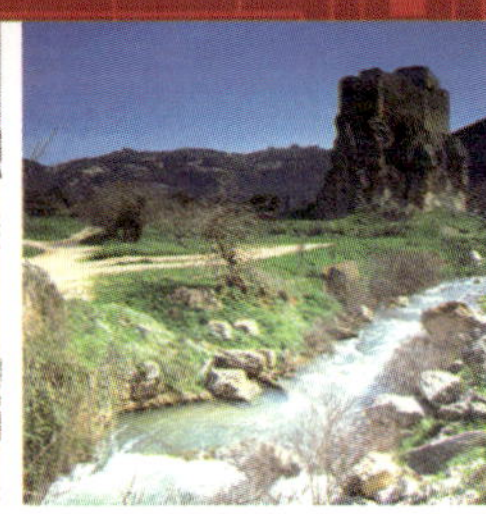
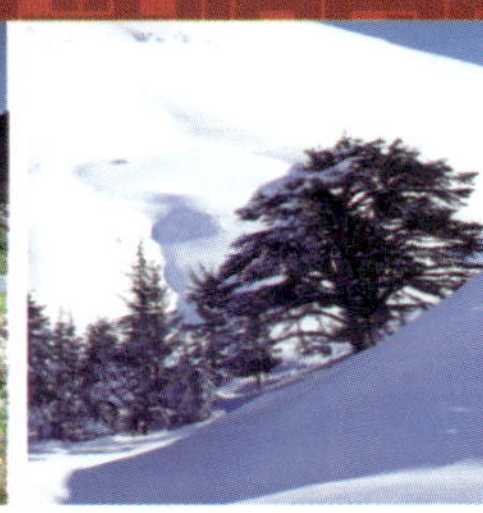
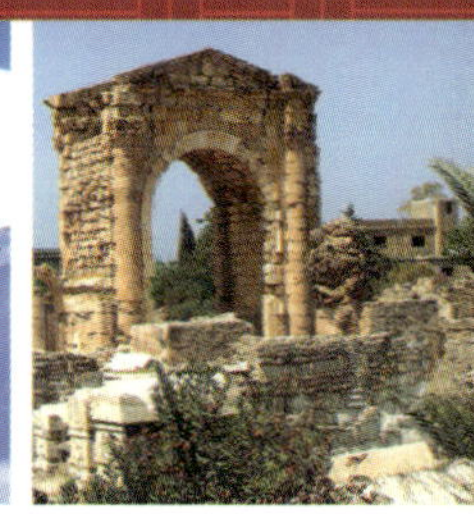

Lebanon is the heart of the Middle East, a unique heart that beats, pushing the people of Lebanon through the country and the Middle East, spreading hospitality, friendship and love all around, still beating since independence was achieved in 1943 and despite years of a recent war. Lebanon remains a small country of a population around 3.5 million and an area of only 10,452 kilometers.

The unique geography of Lebanon portrays a gift from God; sea, mountain, beach, snow and all kinds of entertainment go side-by-side in this ancient country, which has become a great tourist attraction with the ancient Phoenician coastal cities of Beirut, Sidon, Tripoli, Byblos and Tyre.

The Pure Taste of Lebanon from Safa's Kitchen

Printed in the United States of America
First published in 2010 by
The Lebanese Publishing Company
2026 E. Broadway
Tucson, AZ 85719

Text design and layout by Mariam Adra and Nabil Khoury
Photos by John Archuleta
Nutrient analysis by Zeina Makhoul
Editing by Martha Kern

Information in this book is deemed to be authentic and accurate by author and publisher. However, they disclaim any liability incurred in connection with the use of information appearing in this book.

ISBN: 978-0-615-35822-2 (hard back)
1. Cookery, Lebanese. 2. Cookery Middle East. 1. Title

Website: www.safaskitchen.com
E-mail: safa@safaskitchen.com

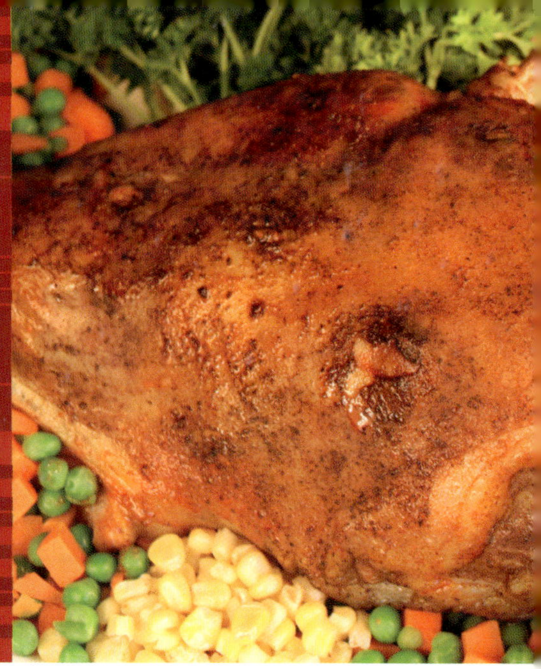

Contents

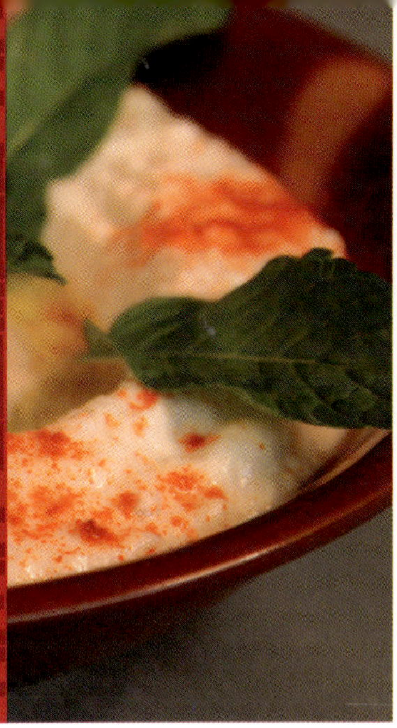 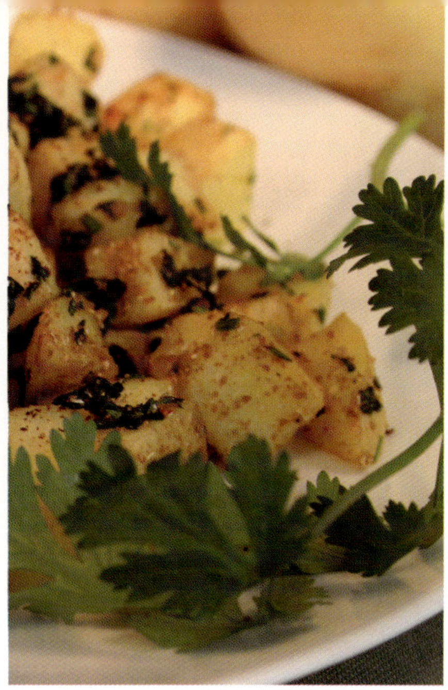 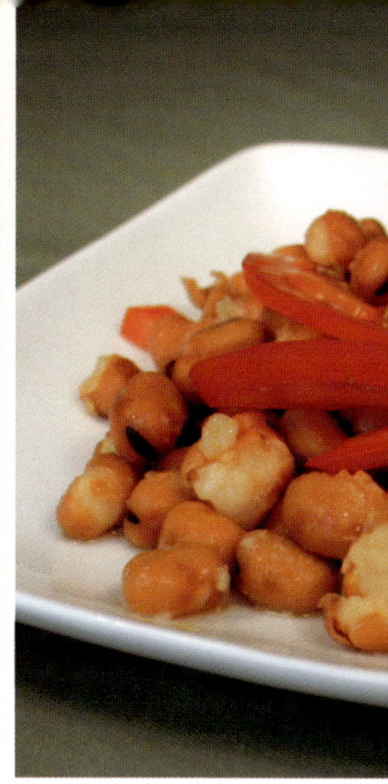

Appetizers: Mezze

المقبلات

There is a Lebanese saying,
"The hands are the keys to the mouth (El yadeyn mfateeh el tim)."

This is an apt description of the traditional Lebanese Mezze, one of the greatest pleasures the country has to offer. Picture a hundred colorful dishes of authentic Mediterranean food accompanied by a hundred different smells, textures and flavors, all to be enjoyed at one sitting. Fresh Arabic bread is an essential tool for hours of sampling the many mouth-watering items at the Mezze – no forks needed here! A licorice-flavored alcoholic drink called arak is common, as well as wine and the nargileh, or water pipe.

The most amazing part of it is that this overwhelming feast is considered merely the appetizer portion of the meal! Some may still order the main course out of courtesy, while others are so full after the Mezze that they pass on the rest of the meal, and top off the evening with fresh fruits and coffee.

This chapter features fifteen common Mezze dishes. Additional recipes that can be used in the Mezze are noted as they appear in other chapters.

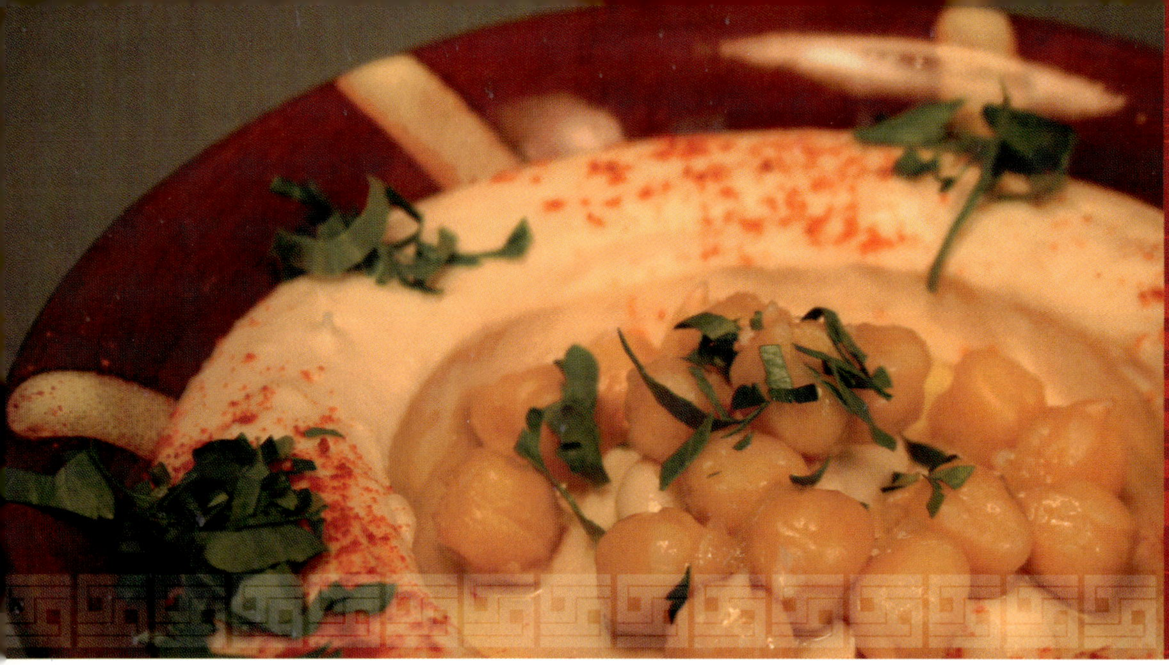

Although convenient hummus dips are available at most supermarkets, making your own is a snap and can help reduce the amount of sodium. If you use canned chick-peas, be sure to rinse them to remove most of the added salt.

Chick-pea Puree: Hummus bi Tahini

حمص بطحينه

Ingredients

2 cups Cooked Chick-peas, drained (reserve liquid)
3 medium garlic cloves, peeled
½ cup sesame seed paste (tahini)
½ teaspoon salt or to taste
¼ cup fresh lemon juice
1 tablespoon extra virgin olive oil

Food processor

Start to Finish
30 minutes
Serves 8

To Garnish

- 1 tablespoon chick-peas
- 1 tablespoon chopped parsley
- ½ teaspoon paprika
- 1 tablespoon extra virgin olive oil

Preparation

Sort and wash 1 cup chick-peas in a colander under cold running water. Soak overnight with 4 cups of water in a heavy pot. The next day, cook over high heat with ½ teaspoon baking soda. Stir and bring to a boil then spoon all the foam from the top and discard. Reduce heat to medium and cook covered for 20 minutes or until soft. Use with any recipe that calls for cooked chick-peas.

Procedure

1• Puree chick-peas and garlic in a food processor.

2• Add sesame seed paste (tahini) and process to blend very well.

3• Add salt and lemon juice and process; add oil and process until puree is creamy. (The thickness of the puree should depend on your taste. If you want to thin it, add more liquid such as 1 tablespoon of liquid reserved from the chick-peas, lemon juice or extra virgin olive oil.)

4• Transfer to a platter, garnish with whole chick-peas and parsley, sprinkle paprika and pour olive oil over it.

Serve it cold or at room temperature with pita bread and pickles.

** TIP This dish can be used as an appetizer, served plain for breakfast, or topped with cooked ground meat and pine nuts for lunch or dinner. It can be reserved in the refrigerator for up to a week.*

Nutrition Information per Serving

Calories 180, Fat 11g, Saturated fat 1.5g, Cholesterol 0mg, Carbohydrate 16g, Fiber 4g, Protein 6.5g

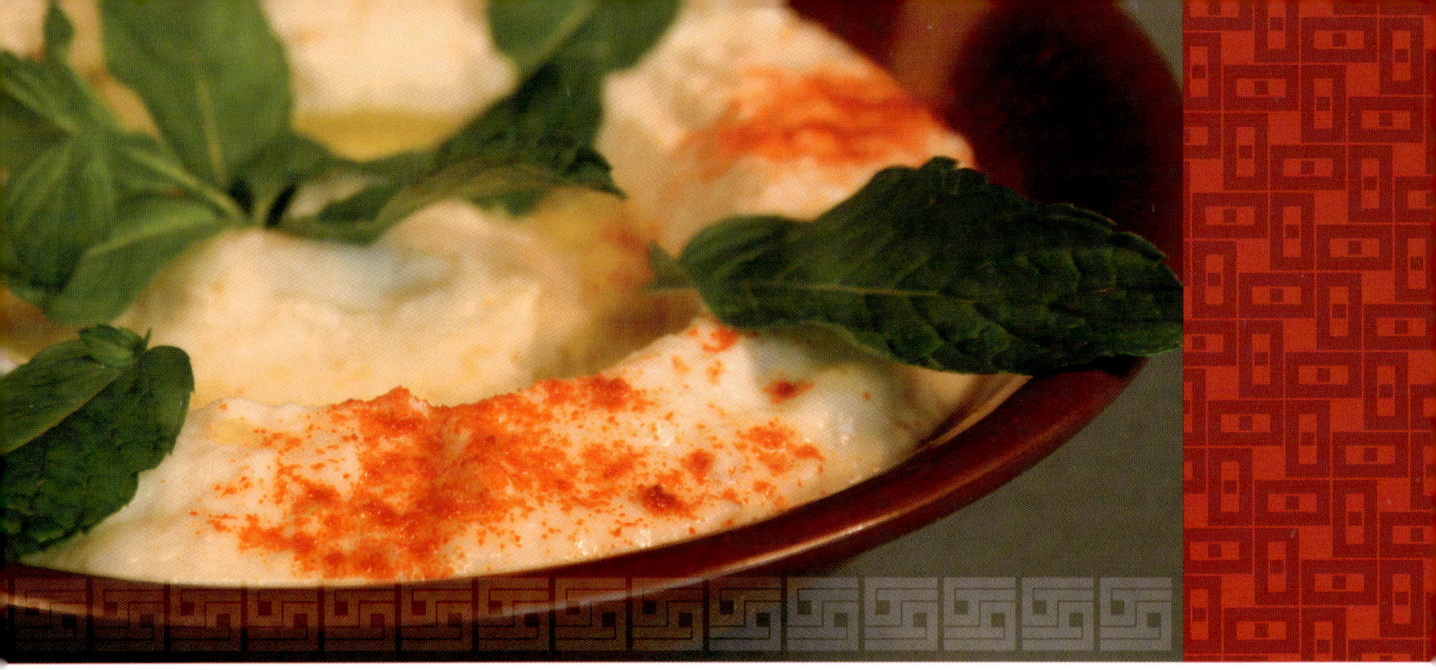

Eggplant Dip: Baba Ghanouj

بابا غنوج

Ingredients

2 large eggplants
2 teaspoons crushed garlic
1 teaspoon salt or to taste
¼ cup fresh lemon juice
¼ cup tahini paste
⅓ cup plain yogurt

Food processor
Toaster oven or oven

Start to Finish
30 minutes
Serves 6

To Garnish

- ¼ teaspoon paprika
- 1 tablespoon finely chopped parsley or a few sprigs of fresh mint
- 2 tablespoons extra virgin olive oil (optional)

Procedure

1• Preheat oven on broil.

2• Poke eggplants 3 times each with a knife and put them in a pan or on a sheet of foil on the bottom rack of the oven. Grill for 20 minutes or until soft, turning those several times to make sure they cook evenly.

3• Once the eggplants are cooled, place them by the kitchen sink and hold each eggplant by the stem then peel under running cold water, then place in a colander to drain. Discard the stems and peels.

4• Place eggplant in a food processor with the garlic and salt and then puree.

5• Transfer pureed mixture into a bowl. Add lemon juice and tahini paste and mix well, and then combine with yogurt.

6• Place dip on a large platter and garnish with paprika, parsley or mint.

Serve it cold with fresh pita bread, pickles and salad, or beside the Kibbeh.

** TIP After cooking and peeling eggplants, sprinkle each with salt to taste and 2 tablespoons fresh lemon juice, and freeze them for up to a month.*

Nutrition Information per Serving

Calories 117, Fat 6g, Saturated fat 1g, Cholesterol 0mg, Carbohydrate 15g, Fiber 5g, Protein 4g

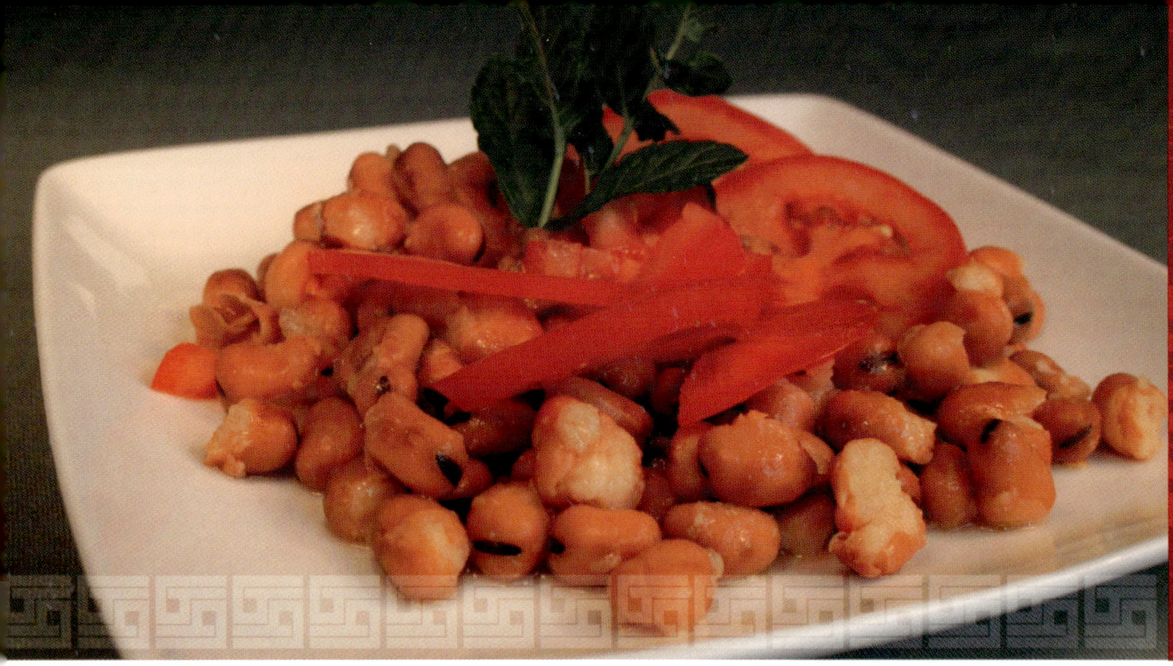

Fava Beans with Garlic & Tomato:

Fool M'dammas

فول مدمس

Ingredients

One 15-oz. can fava beans
3 medium cloves garlic, peeled and crushed
¼ cup fresh lemon juice
½ teaspoon salt or to taste
¼ cup extra virgin olive oil
1 large tomato, finely diced
Mint leaves

Fresh pita bread
1 onion, quartered and soaked in ice water
Fresh radishes

Start to Finish
15 minutes
Serves 2

To Garnish

- ¼ teaspoon paprika
- 1 tablespoon finely chopped parsley or a few sprigs of fresh mint
- 2 tablespoons extra virgin olive oil (optional)

Procedure

1• Place fava beans in a saucepan with ½ cup water, bring to a boil over high heat for 10 minutes and set aside.

2• Put garlic, lemon juice and salt in a bowl and stir, then add olive oil.

3• With a potato masher or a pestle, partially smash the fava beans and add them to the lemon mixture. Add diced tomato, reserving 1 tablespoon for a garnish.

4• Fold to combine and transfer to a large platter. Decorate the top with the diced tomato and mint leaves, and then serve.

Serve it hot, warm or cold with fresh pita bread, onion, radishes and pickles, for breakfast, lunch or dinner or as an appetizer.

** TIP Leftover bean mixture refrigerates well up to a week. If you like cooked chick-peas, add 1 cup to the fava beans for a delicious combination.*

Nutrition Information per Serving

Calories 691, Fat 38g, Saturated fat 11g, Cholesterol 22mg, Carbohydrate 65g, Fiber 17.5g, Protein 24g

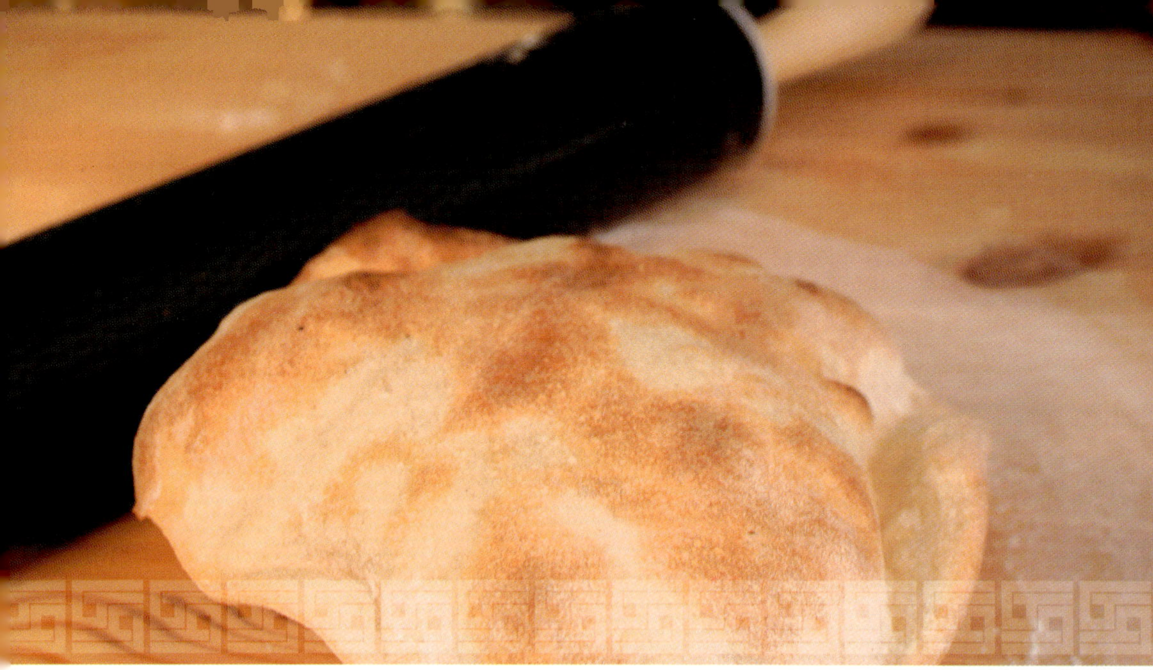

Pita Bread: Khobz Arabi

خبز عربي

Dough Ingredients

1 teaspoon active dry yeast
¼ teaspoon sugar
1¼ cups warm water
3 cups all-purpose flour
½ teaspoon salt

Electric food processor
Rolling pin
Flour
Aluminum foil

Start to Finish
20 minutes
plus resting time.

Procedure

1• Stir 1 teaspoon active dry yeast into ¼ cup warm water, then stir in ¼ teaspoon sugar. Let stand for 5 minutes.

2• Meanwhile, put flour and salt in the food processor and mix briefly.

3• With food processor running, slowly add yeast mixture and 1 cup warm water through a feed tube to make dough stick together and form a ball, about 40 seconds. You might need to add 1 more tablespoon of warm water. The dough should be a bit soft but not sticky.

4• Turn dough onto a floured surface and knead by hand about 5 turns. This will make finely-textured dough.

5• Divide dough equally into 8 parts, cover, and let it rest in a warm place until it doubles in size (about 1 hour). After the dough has risen, punch each part down with your hands and form it into a rough round shape. Let it rest for 5 minutes.

6• Line the oven racks with sheets of foil and heat oven to 500 degrees F.

7• With a rolling pin, roll a piece of dough on a floured surface into a 1/8-inch thick circle that is about 8 inches in diameter. Set aside on a floured surface.

8• Roll out the remaining dough in the same way. Sprinkle the rolling pin and rolling surface regularly with flour so the dough will not stick.

9• Open the oven. Slide out the first rack and transfer as many rounds as will fit on it. Place the remaining rounds on the other racks.

10• Close the oven and bake them for 3 minutes or until the bread rises and turns a light golden color. Remove rounds from oven and cool for 5 minutes. Place them in a plastic bag so they will stay fresh.

Serve hot, fresh from the oven, or warm with food of your choice.

** TIP Baked bread and leftover dough freeze well in an airtight bag.*

Nutrition Information per Serving

Calories 162, Fat 0g, Saturated fat 0g, Cholesterol 0mg, Carbohydrate 34g, Fiber 2g, Protein 6g

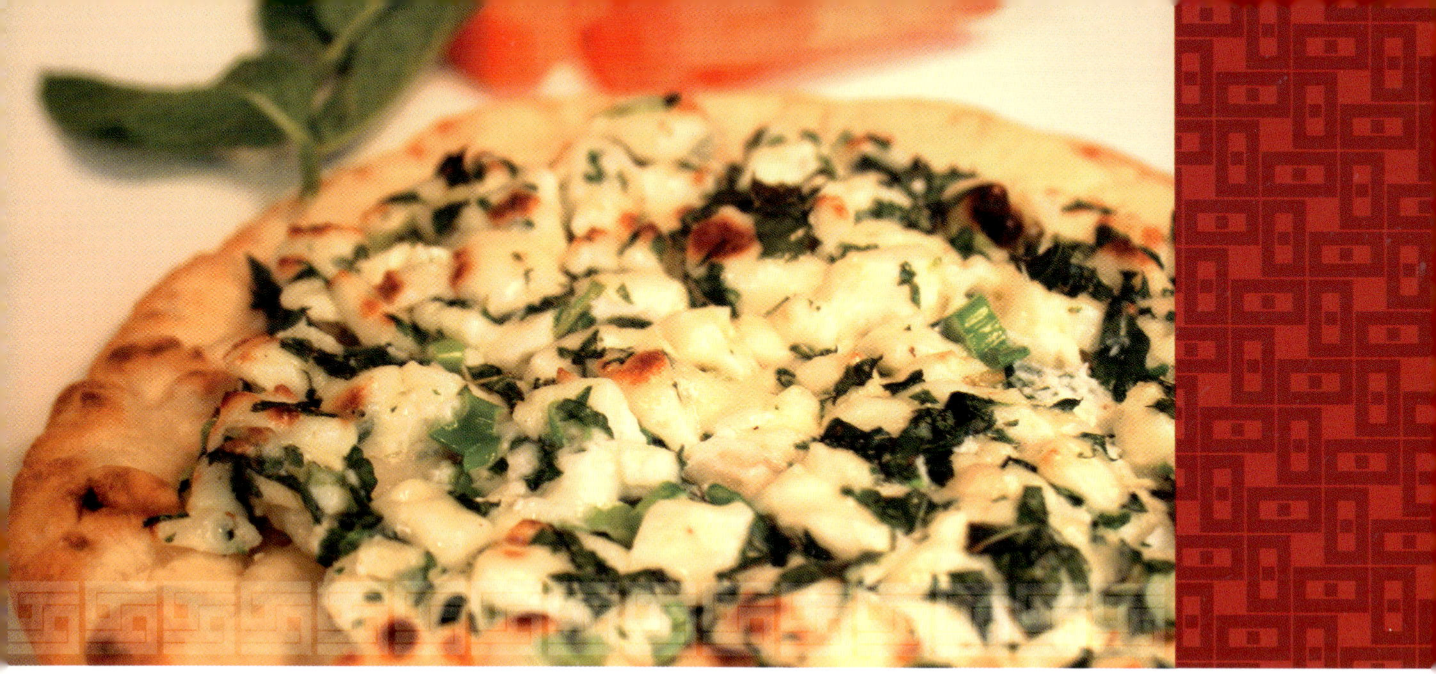

Lebanese Cheese Tart: Mana'eesh b'Jebin

مناقيش بجبن

Ingredients

1 recipe Pita Bread dough divided into 8 parts
1½ pounds feta cheese or akkawi cheese, shredded
¾ cup finely chopped fresh mint
½ cup finely chopped scallions
1 large egg white
½ teaspoon salt
¼ teaspoon ground black pepper
1 tablespoon olive oil

Aluminum foil to line the oven racks OR
Cookie sheets

Start to Finish
20 minutes
plus prepared dough

Preparation

Pita Bread dough prepared and set aside

Procedure

1• Line oven racks with aluminum foil or place cookie sheets in oven.

2• Preheat oven to 500 degrees F.

3• Mix together all ingredients except bread dough and set aside.

4• Roll each of the 8 dough pieces into a 1/8-inch round on a floured counter. Press down each piece with your fingers so the dough will not swell when you bake it. Spread 2 tablespoons cheese mixture on each round to make a pie, leaving ¼ inch empty around the edge

5• Sprinkle a large, flat platter with flour. Place one uncooked cheese tart on the platter, and then slide the tart onto the hot, foil-lined oven rack or onto a heated cookie sheet.

6• Transfer remaining tarts in the same way and bake them for 5 minutes or until golden.

Serve it hot or warm for breakfast or lunch, or as an appetizer.

***TIP Cheese tarts freeze well in an airtight plastic bag.**

*** You can also use ready-made dough from any Middle Eastern grocery store.**

Nutrition Information per Serving

Calories 209, Fat 10g, Saturated fat 6g, Cholesterol 38mg, Carbohydrate 20g, Fiber 1g, Protein 9g

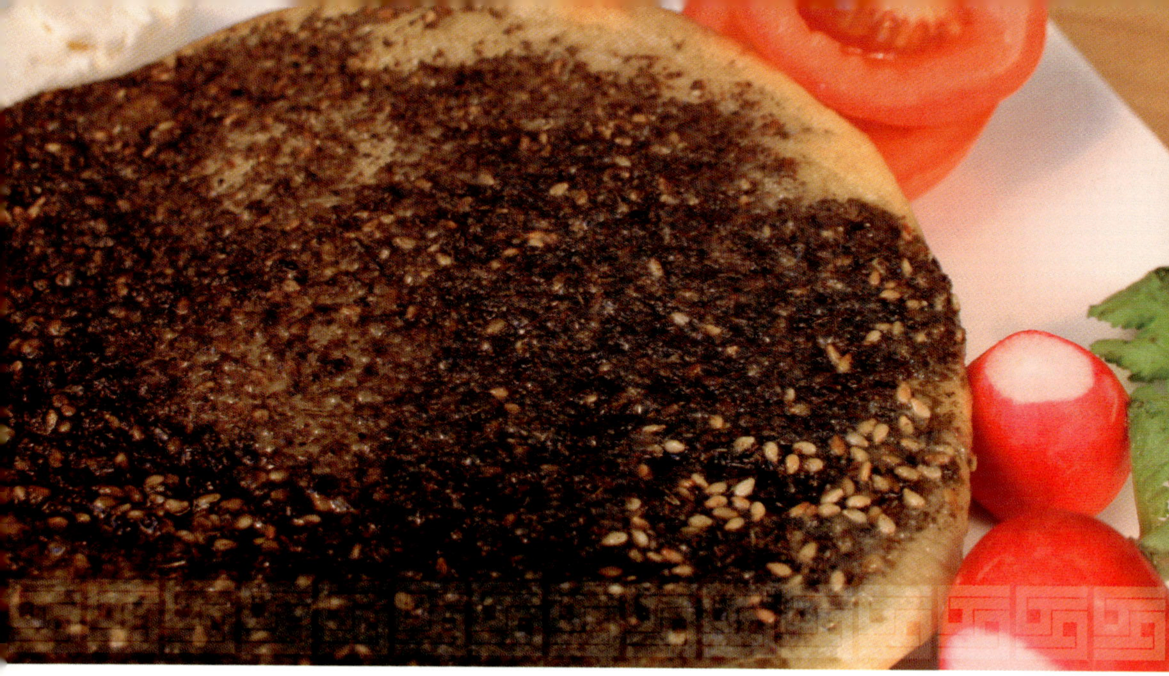

Preparing Mana'eesh is fun. You get to play with the dough after rolling it out by gently punching it with your fingers, so the tart will not swell when you bake it.
Mana'eesh is usually topped with a zaa'tar mixture, which is a combination of thyme, sesame seeds and dried sumac with olive oil, but it can be topped with cheese, meat or another favorite topping.

Lebanese Thyme Tart: Mana'eesh b'Zaa'tar

مناقيش بزعتر

Ingredients

1 recipe Pita Bread dough divided into 8 parts
(See Lebanese cheese tart)
4 tablespoons Zaa'tar
4 tablespoons extra virgin olive oil

Aluminum foil to line the oven racks OR
Cookie sheets

Start to Finish
20 minutes
plus bread dough

Preparation

Pita Bread dough prepared and set aside

Procedure

1• Cover oven racks with aluminum foil or place cookie sheets in cold oven.

2• Preheat oven to 500 degrees F.

3• Mix Zaa'tar and oil and set aside.

4• Roll out each piece of dough into a 1/8-inch thick round on a floured surface. Punch the dough with your fingers and spread one tablespoon Zaa'tar mixture on the surface, leaving ¼ inch empty around the edges.

5• Sprinkle a large, flat platter with flour. Place one uncooked tart on the platter and slide it onto one of the hot oven racks or onto a heated cookie sheet.

6• Transfer remaining tarts in the same way and bake for 5 minutes or until golden in color.

Serve it hot or warm as a sandwich for breakfast, as a snack with tea and orange juice or as a light dinner.

** TIP Mana'eesh will freeze well up to 2 months in an airtight bag or in a covered container.*

Nutrition Information per Serving

Calories 129, Fat 5g, Saturated fat 1g, Cholesterol 0mg, Carbohydrate 19g, Fiber 1g, Protein 3g

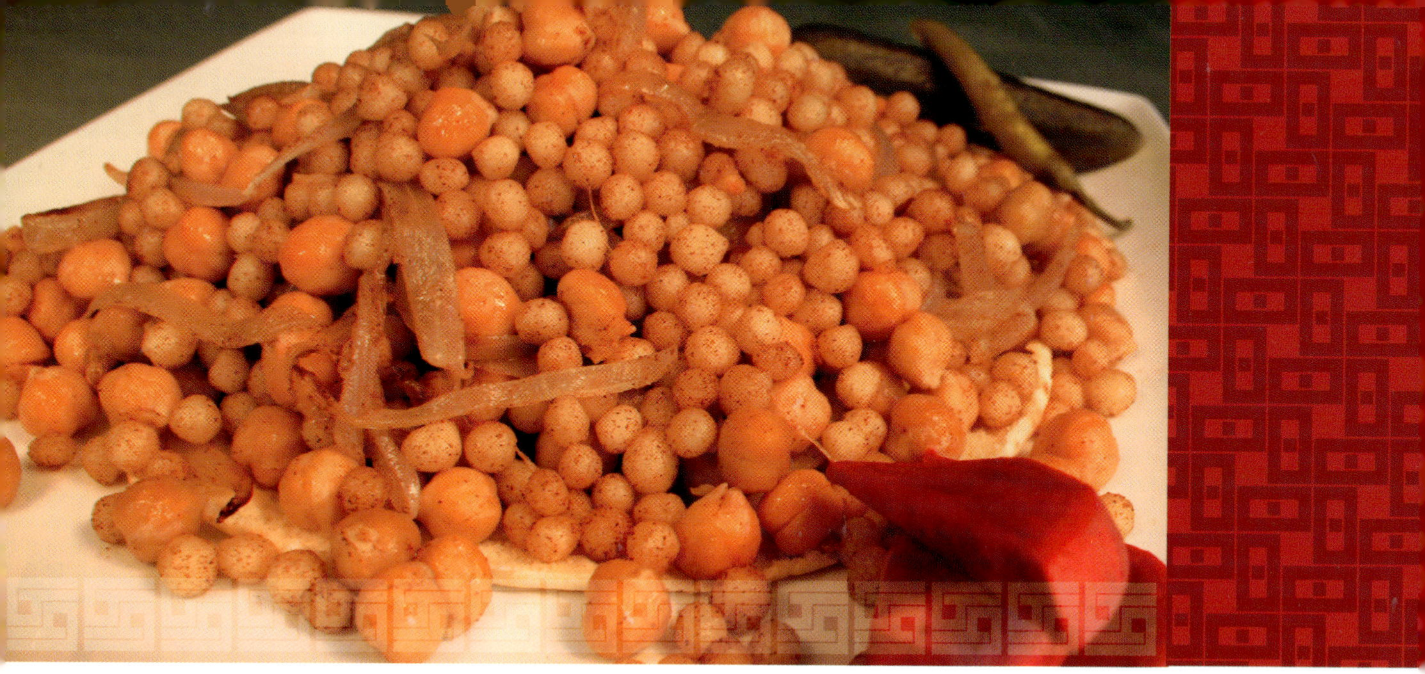

Lebanese Couscous: Moghrabieh

مغربية

Ingredients

16 oz. Mograbieh (dried couscous)
2 medium onion sliced into ⅛ - inch wedges
15 oz. can of chick-peas, rinsed and drained
1 teaspoon salt or to taste
1 teaspoon cinnamon

¼ cup clarified butter
Fresh pita bread
Turnip and cucumber pickles

Start to Finish
30 minutes
Serves 8

Preparation

- Bring 4 to 6 quarts of water to a rapid boil over high heat. If desired, add 1 to 2 teaspoons of salt.
- Add dried couscous to boiling water, stirring occasionally.
- Cook for 12 minutes or until desired degree of tenderness is reached.

Drain and set aside.

Procedure

1• Meanwhile, place clarified butter in a large skillet over medium-high heat to melt, add onion and sauté for few minutes to wilt.

2• Add chick-peas and sauté for several minutes, then reduce heat to medium and cook covered for 5 minutes.

3• Uncover the skillet and add the drained couscous, stir to combine and sauté for 5 minutes.

4• Sprinkle with salt and combine. Sprinkle cinnamon all over couscous mixture, combine well and cook for several more minutes.

5• Open one pita round and place it on a platter. Turn off the heat and transfer cooked couscous onto the platter lined with the bread. Open another pita and place it on top of the couscous to keep it moist until it is served.

Serve it hot or warm with fresh bread and Turnip Pickles for breakfast. For lunch or dinner you can add cooked chicken pieces and broth, sauté for few minutes and then serve.

** TIP Lebanese Couscous is a simple, delicious dish for a buffet. If this recipe is too large, you can freeze half of the couscous before you sauté it, and keep it up to 3 months.*

Nutrition Information per Serving

Calories 414, Fat 9g, Saturated fat 4g, Cholesterol 14mg, Carbohydrate 71g, Fiber 6.5g, Protein 13g

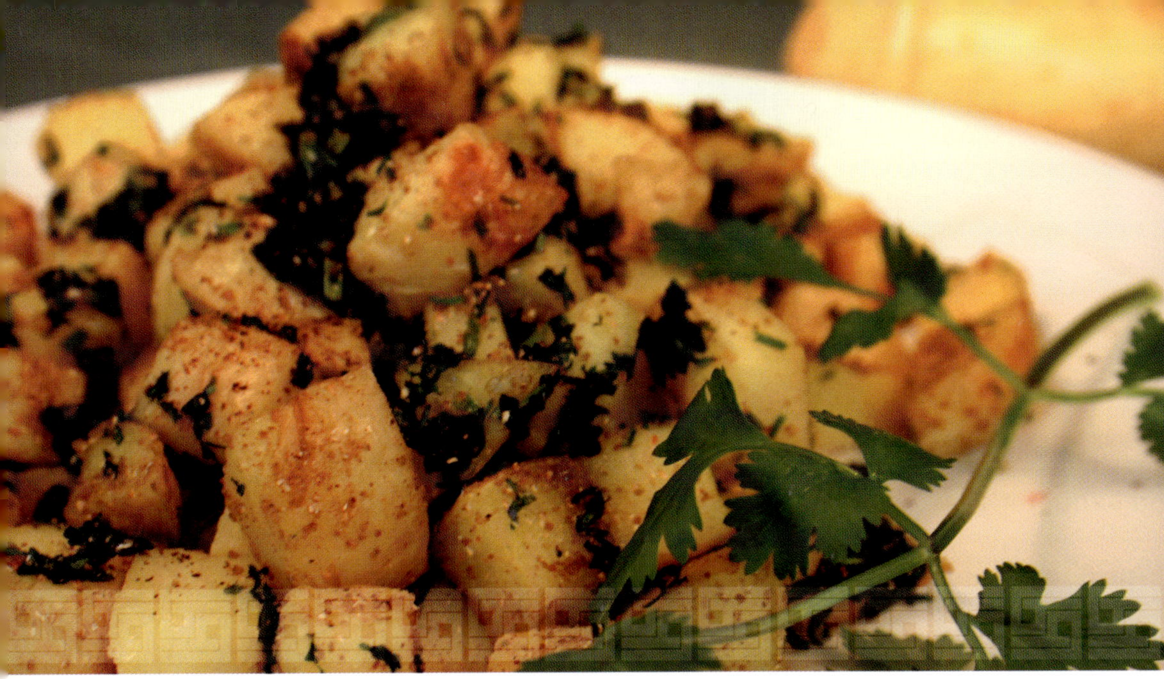

Potatoes with Cilantro: Batata b' Kizibra

بطاطا بكزبره

Ingredients

4 medium potatoes, peeled and diced into 1-inch cubes
¼ cup oil
1 packed cup chopped cilantro
1 teaspoon crushed garlic
½ teaspoon salt
1 teaspoon ground coriander
1 tablespoon sumac (optional)

Large skillet

Start to Finish
25 minutes
Serves 4

Procedure

1• Place oil in the skillet over medium heat, add diced potatoes and cook covered for 10 minutes.

2• Remove lid from skillet, stir well, then replace lid and cook for 10 more minutes or until soft, stirring twice.

3• Add chopped cilantro and garlic, stir, and cook briefly, then sprinkle with salt, coriander and sumac and mix well. Turn off heat, transfer to a platter and serve.

Serve it hot or warm as an appetizer.

** TIP This dish tastes better when it is fresh. Diced potatoes can be deep fried then sautéed with the remaining ingredients.*

Nutrition Information per Serving

Calories 184, Fat 7g, Saturated fat 1g, Cholesterol 0mg, Carbohydrate 29g, Fiber 3g, Protein 3g

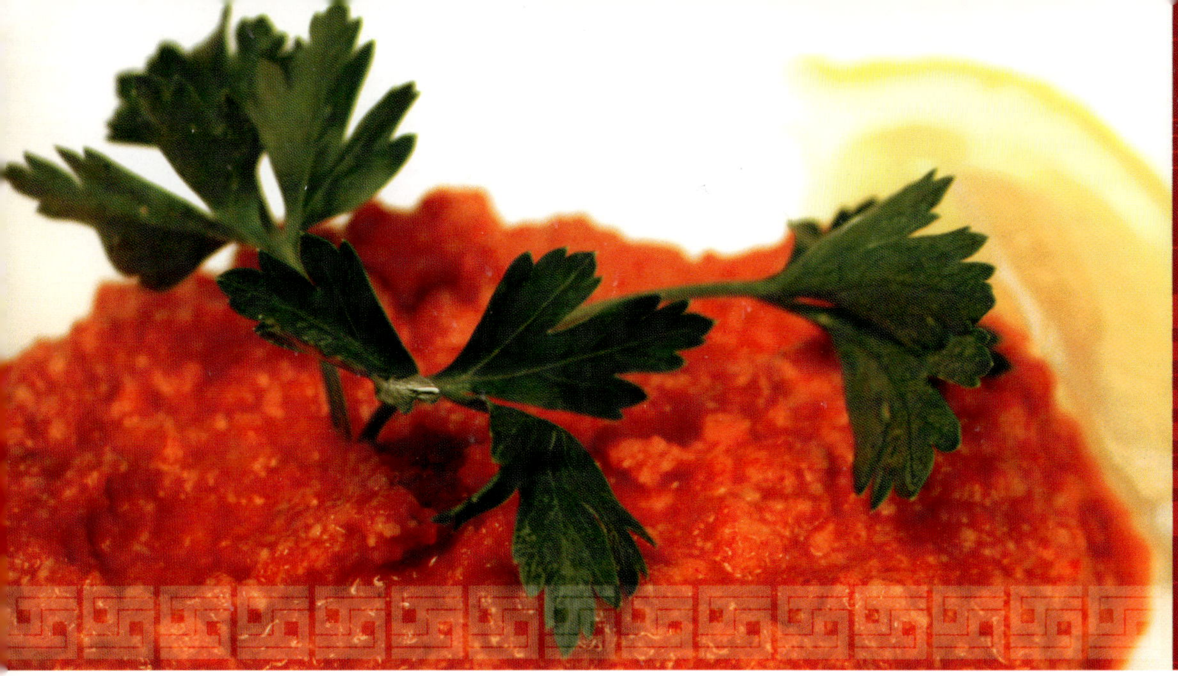

Red Pepper Puree: M'hamra

محمره

Ingredients

2 large red peppers, quartered
1 small onion, quartered
½ teaspoon salt or to taste
2 tablespoons fresh lemon juice
½ teaspoon sugar
½ cup bread crumbs
½ cup ground walnuts
1 tablespoon extra virgin olive oil

Food processor

Start to Finish
7 minutes
Serves 6

To Garnish

• Mint leaves or parsley
• Lemon wedges

Procedure

1• Puree red pepper and onion in a food processor until smooth.

2• Add salt and lemon juice, process to mix, then transfer to a bowl.

3• Stir in sugar, then add bread crumbs, walnuts, olive oil and mix well.

4• Transfer to a platter and garnish with mint or parsley.

Serve it cold or at room temperature with pita bread as an appetizer dish.

** TIP If you like it hot, add ½ teaspoon crushed red pepper or to taste; or, if you like the flavor of cumin add ½ teaspoon. Chili can be used instead of red pepper.*

Nutrition Information per Serving

Calories 95, Fat 7g, Saturated fat 1g, Cholesterol 0mg, Carbohydrate 8g, Fiber 2g, Protein 2g

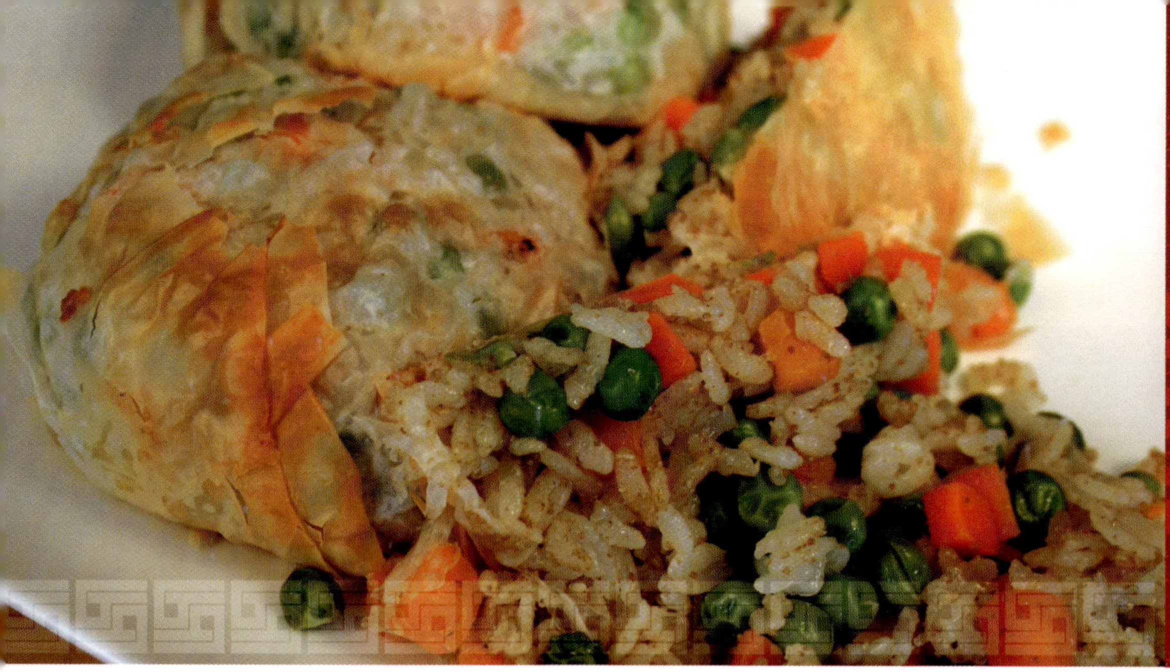

Imagine yourself walking down the street past a bakery when you are drawn inside the shop by the inviting aroma of freshly-baked bread or pie. The same thing will happen at home when you bake savory pastries– family members will come running and pretend to help, but what they really want is to sample those fragrant morsels as they come out of the oven. Savory pastries are extremely popular in Lebanon, and are served at every buffet and birthday party, as well as for a light lunch or as part of the hot Mezze. In this recipe you are going to learn how to fill the ready-made phyllo dough with vegetables and rice and in the next recipe you will learn how to make homemade dough.

Rice and Vegetable Pie: Ouzi

اوزي

Ingredients

2 cups cooked Plain Rice
2 cups frozen mixed vegetables, thawed
¼ teaspoon ground seven spices
½ teaspoon coriander
½ teaspoon salt
8 sheets frozen phyllo dough, thawed
1 deep soup cup (4 ¼ x 3 inches)
¼ cup clarified butter or vegetable oil

Pastry brush
Medium-sized greased pan

Start to Finish
30 minutes
Serves 4

Preparation

- Cooked Plain Rice prepared and set aside
- Thaw vegetables to room temperature
- Thaw phyllo dough to room temperature

Procedure

1• Heat oven to 450 degrees F.

2• Mix rice, vegetables and spices in a large bowl.

3• Place 1 sheet phyllo dough on a work surface. Brush half the phyllo with butter and fold it. Gently place it in the soup cup as a liner, with the sides hanging on the sides of the cup.

4• Put 1 cup filling in the soup cup over the phyllo.
Fold the sides over the filling to close and brush the top with butter.

5• Place another sheet of phyllo dough on the work surface and brush it with butter. Gently invert the filled dough that is in the soup cup over the phyllo sheet. Fold the phyllo sheet and wrap it around the filled dough, forming a ball shape. Brush the ball with butter and place it in the pan seam side down.

6• Finish the remaining sheets in the same way and bake for 10 minutes, turning them once after 7 minutes.

Serve it hot with plain yogurt and salad.

** TIP Plain rice can be prepared a few days in advance. Meat lovers can add one cup meat with pine nuts to the filling, which can also be prepared several days ahead.*

Nutrition Information per Serving

Calories 640, Fat 17g, Saturated fat 2g, Cholesterol 0mg, Carbohydrate 106g, Fiber 7g, Protein 14g

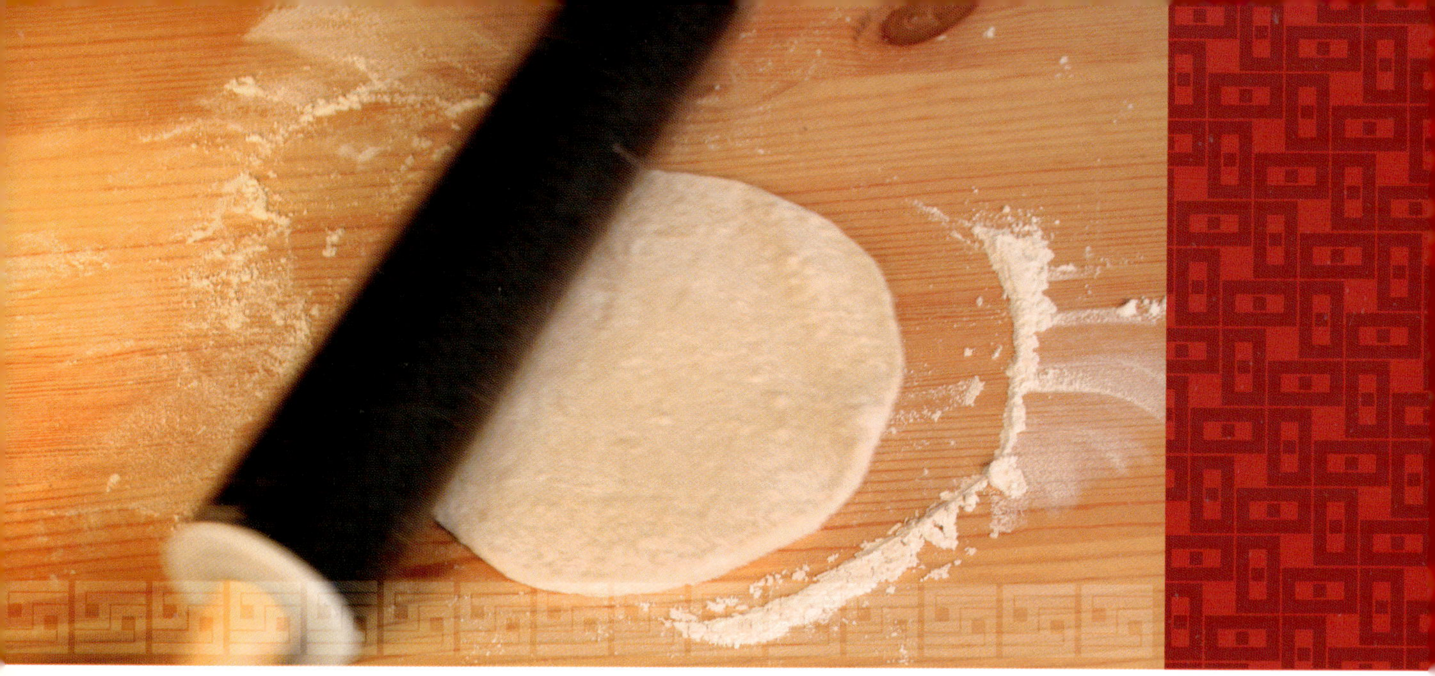

Spinach Pie Dough: Ajeenet el Sabanikh

عجينه السبانخ

Ingredients

1 teaspoon active dry yeast
1 teaspoon sugar
1 cup warm water
3 cups all-purpose flour
1 teaspoon salt
¼ cup olive oil

Start to Finish
5 minutes plus resting time

Procedure

1• Put yeast and sugar in a small bowl with warm water, stir, and set aside for several minutes to rise.

2• Place flour and salt in the food processor and process for 5 seconds.

3• With the processor running, pour in oil through a feeding tube. Slowly add yeast mixture and process until dough sticks together and forms a ball, about 1 minute.

4• Turn out dough onto a floured surface and knead it by hand about 5 turns until smooth in texture.

5• Split the dough into halves and place them apart on a large platter. Cover, and let them rise in a warm place until they double in size, about 1 hour.

* *TIP Leftover dough can be refrigerated for several days or frozen for 1 month.*

Nutrition Information per Serving

Calories 124, Fat 4g, Saturated fat 1g, Cholesterol 0mg, Carbohydrate 19g, Fiber 1g, Protein 3g

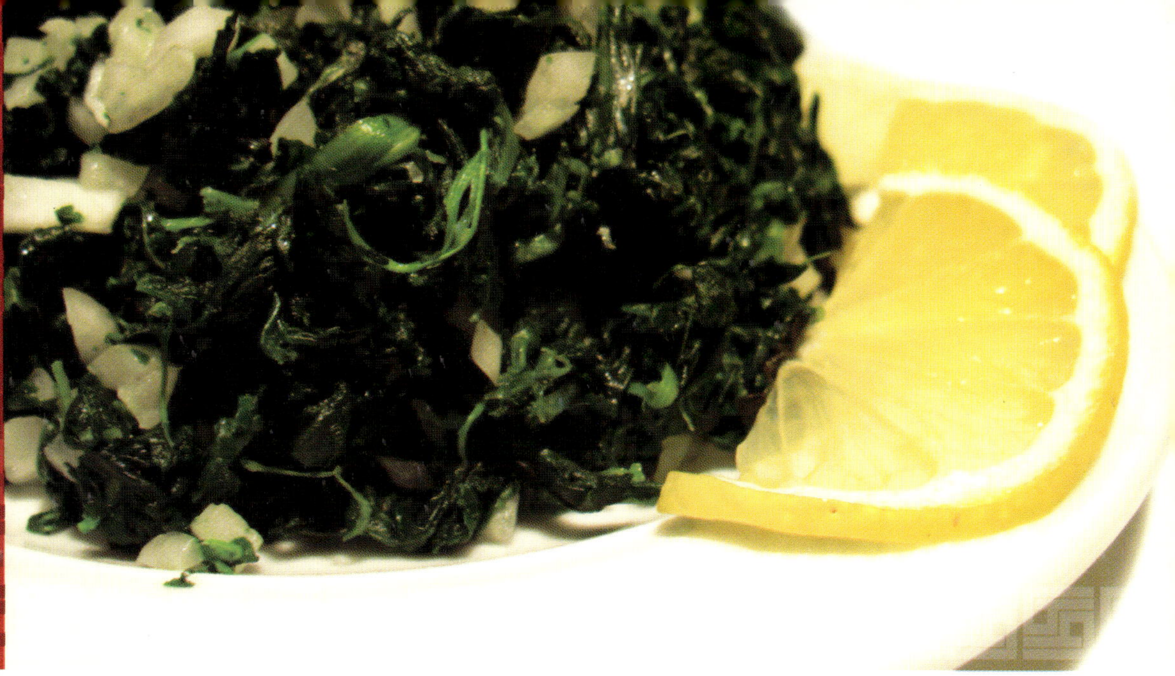

Spinach with Onion: Hashwet el Sabanekh

حشوة السبانخ

Ingredients

1 pound frozen chopped baby spinach thawed
1 medium onion, finely chopped
1 teaspoon salt
¼ teaspoon ground black pepper
¼ cup lemon juice
2 tablespoons olive oil

Start to Finish
15 minutes

Procedure

1• Squeeze spinach in a sifter to get rid of all the water and place in a bowl.

2• Place chopped onion on a plate, sprinkle salt over it, smash it well with your fingers then add it to the spinach and mix to combine.

3• Add the remaining ingredient one at a time and stir well to combine..

** TIP Use this filling with any dough, bread or croissant. You can even add 1 cup walnut broken into little pieces.*

Nutrition Information per Serving

Calories 27, Fat 2g, Saturated fat 0g, Cholesterol 0mg, Carbohydrate 2g, Fiber 1g, Protein 1g

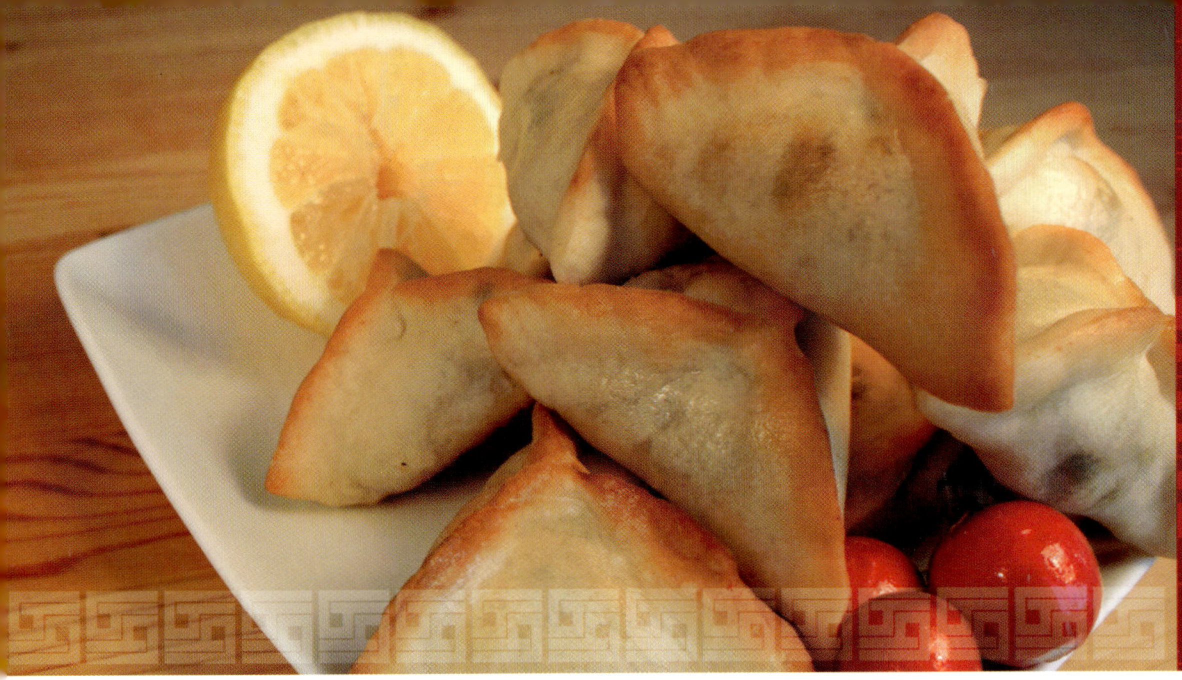

Spinach Pie: Fatayer b'Sabanikh

فطاير بسبانخ

Ingredients

1 recipe Spinach Pie Dough
1 recipe Spinach with Onion filling

¼ cup flour to roll out dough
3-inch round cookie cutter
Two 12 x 14-inch pans
Heat oven to 500 F.

Start to Finish
1 hour
plus prepared dough
Makes 60 pies
Serves 15

Preparation

- Spinach Pie Dough prepared and set aside (see page 28)
- Spinach with Onion filling prepared and set aside (see page 29)

Procedure

1• Roll out dough with a rolling pin on a lightly flowered surface to the thickness of less than ⅛ inch.

2• Cut dough with 3-inch round cookie cutter. Gather trimmings into a ball and cover with plastic to rest.

3• Turn the dough circles upside down. Place 1 tablespoon spinach filling in the middle of each round. Be careful to keep the filling away from the edges, as this will make it easier to seal them closed.

4• Hold a round in the palm of your left hand and press lightly on the filling with your thumb. With 3 fingers from your right hand (thumb, pointer, middle), gather the edges of the dough to close the pie and form a triangle. (Use opposite hands if you are left-handed). Press well on the 3 sides and place it on the cookie sheet.

5• Follow this process to finish all rounds and the rest of the dough.

6• Bake for 5 minutes, then turn the pans and bake for 2 more minutes or until golden brown.

Serve it warm or cold as an appetizer with lemon wedges.

** TIP Filling may be prepared a few days in advance. Dough and pies freeze well for up to 2 months.*

Nutrition Information per Serving

Calories 151, Fat 6g, Saturated fat 1g, Cholesterol 0mg, Carbohydrate 21g, Fiber 2g, Protein 4g

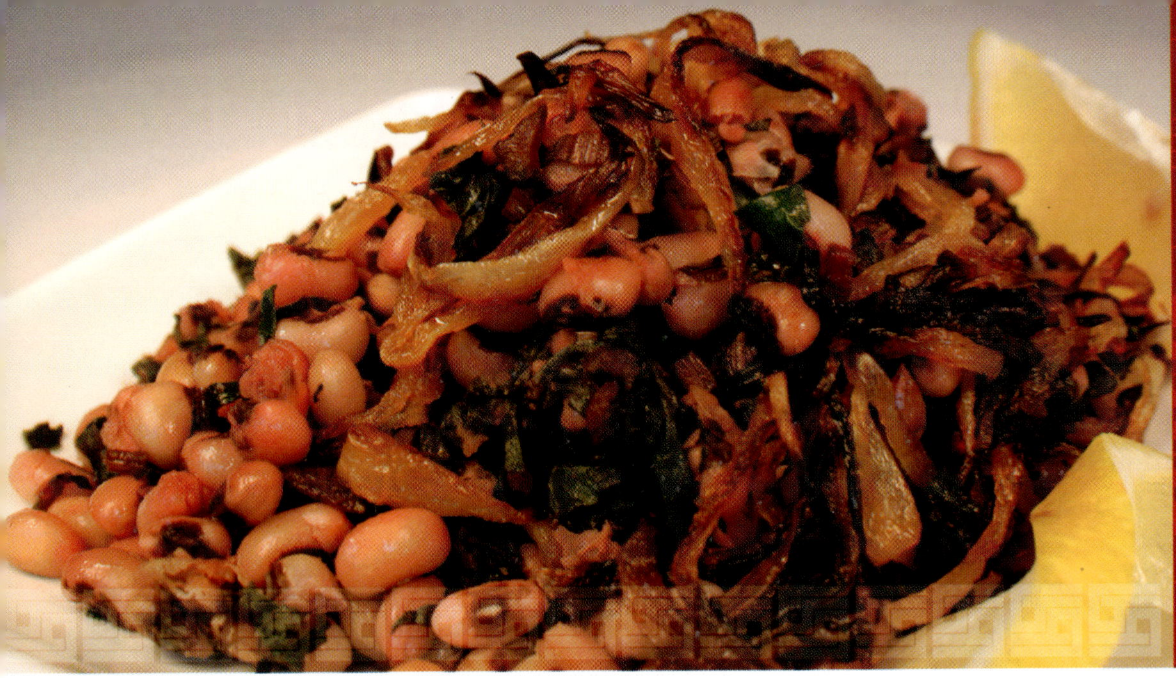

Swiss Chard with Black-eyed Peas:

Silik b'Loubieh

سلق بلوبيه

Ingredients

10 oz. frozen black-eyed peas, thawed
1 bunch Swiss chard, washed and finely chopped
3 cups water
⅓ cup olive oil
1 large onion sliced in ⅛ -inch wedges
1 bunch cilantro, washed and finely chopped
1 tablespoon minced garlic
1 teaspoon salt
¼ teaspoon ground black pepper

Large skillet
Paper towel

Start to Finish
30 minutes
Serves 6

Procedure

1• Place black-eyed peas in a large skillet with 3 cups water.
Boil on high heat for 7 minutes.

2• Stir in Swiss chard and bring to a boil again, then reduce heat to medium and cook covered for 15 minutes, stirring occasionally.

3• Meanwhile, pour oil in a large pan, stir in onion wedges and sauté until golden brown. Remove wedges with a slotted spoon onto a plate lined with paper towels to drain. Save hot oil in the pan.

4• Sauté chopped cilantro and garlic in hot oil over medium-high heat for 1 minute, then add mixture with the oil to the chard skillet. Sprinkle salt and pepper, combine well, and cook 5 more minutes or until soft.

5• Turn off heat and let food sit for a few minutes. Transfer cooked Swiss chard to a large platter, garnish the top with the cooked onion and serve.

Serve it warm or at room temperature with fresh pita bread, radishes, scallions, salad and fresh lemon wedges to squeeze over the Swiss chard.

** TIP This dish can be server as an appetizer.*

Nutrition Information per Serving

Calories 182, Fat 12g, Saturated fat 2g, Cholesterol 0mg, Carbohydrate 15g, Fiber 4g, Protein 5g

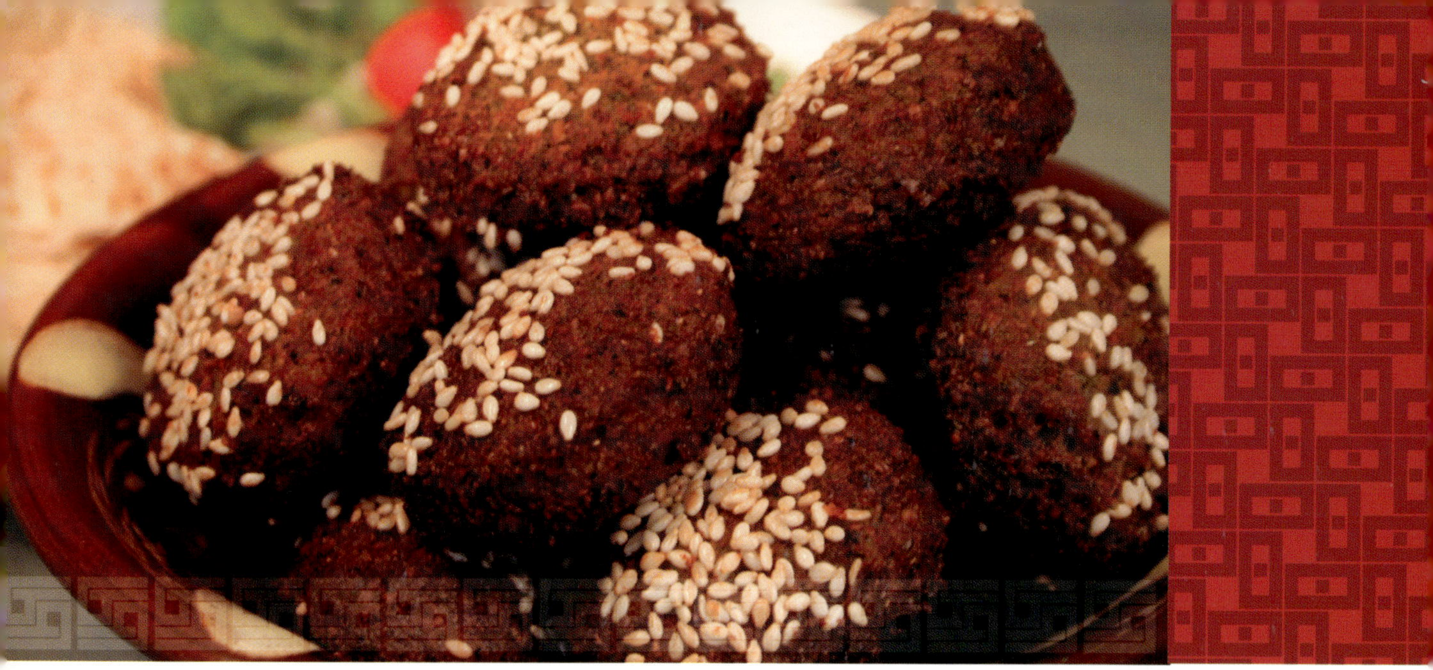

Vegetarian Patties: Falafel

فلافل

Ingredients

¼ cup chick-peas (soaked overnight)
¾ cup peeled fava beans (soaked overnight)
1 cup packed cilantro, trimmed and washed
¼ cup packed parsley, trimmed and washed
1 small onion, peeled and quartered
4 fresh garlic cloves, peeled
½ teaspoon ground cumin
1 teaspoon ground coriander
1 teaspoon salt
½ teaspoon baking soda

Start to Finish
25 minutes
plus soaking time
Serves 6

Food processor
2 tablespoons sesame seeds
Falafel scoop or a tablespoon
Deep fryer pan
Vegetable oil

Preparation

- The night before, soak chick-peas and fava beans together in three times their volume of water, as they double in size.

Tahini Sauce: Tarator

½ cup tahini paste, ½ cup water, ¼ cup lemon juice, 1 teaspoon crushed garlic and 1 teaspoon salt. Put tahini paste in a bowl and gradually pour in water while stirring. Add lemon juice, garlic and salt, and blend until smooth.

Procedure

1• The next day, rinse the beans and drain.
Transfer onto a platter lined with paper towels and pat dry.

2• Pat dry cilantro and parsley then place beans, cilantro, parsley, onion, garlic, cumin, coriander, salt and baking soda in a food processor and process into a very fine mixture.

3• Transfer falafel mixture into a bowl, sprinkle sesame seeds over the top and start shaping the mixture. Scoop a tablespoon of the mixture and level it by sliding a dull knife on the surface of the spoon.

4• With the tip of a knife, slide patty off the spoon onto a large platter.
(Dipping the empty spoon into a half filled cup of water before each use and shaking off the excess water will make it easier to slide the patties off the spoon.)
Continue shaping the mixture, you will have 24 patties.

5• In a deep fryer pot, heat about 2 inches oil to 400 degrees F. (Oil should be very hot before adding patties). Gently lift and drop in falafel patties one at a time, as many as will comfortably fit. Fry on both sides until golden brown.

6• Remove patties with a slotted spoon and place them on a platter layered with paper towels to drain excess oil.

7• Fry remaining falafel patties and serve them hot.

Serve Falafel hot or warm with pita bread as an appetizer or as a Falafel sandwich for lunch or dinner with turnips, cucumbers, hot pepper pickles, diced tomatoes, chopped parsley and tahini sauce.

** TIP Heat the oil while you are shaping the patties.*
Or, patties can be covered and refrigerated for a couple of days before frying.

Nutrition Information per Serving

Calories 256, Fat 10.5g, Saturated fat 1g, Cholesterol 0mg, Carbohydrate 31g, Fiber 9.5g, Protein 10.5g

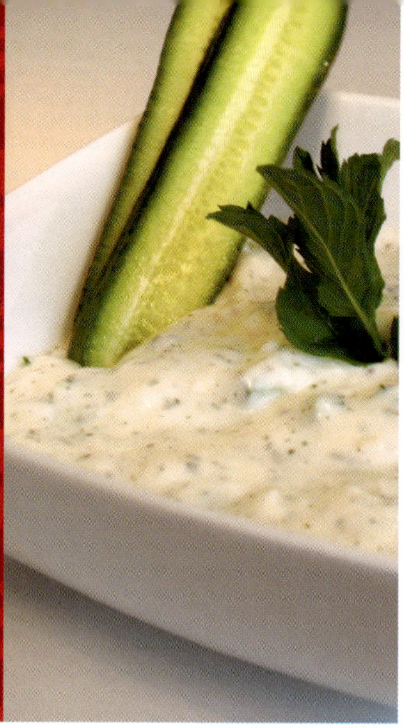 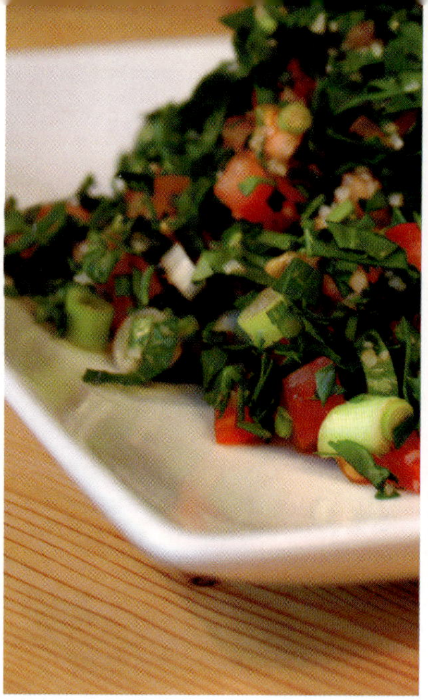 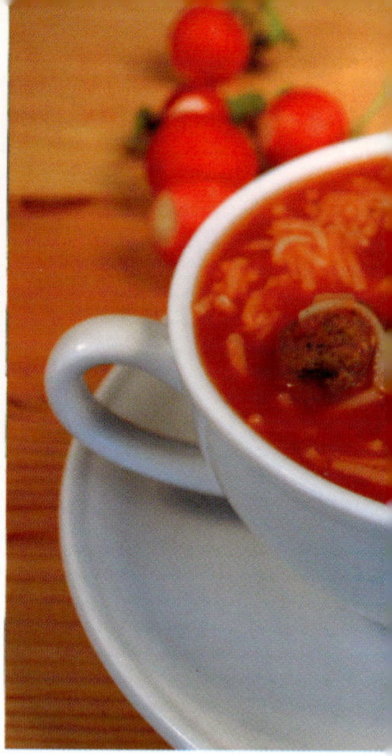

Salads and Soups: El Salatat wal shorbat

السلطات والشوربات

Colorful and nutritious salads topped with lemon-garlic dressing and cold-pressed extra virgin olive oil are shared in this chapter, as well as light meal in the summer. They are enjoyed by children and grown-ups alike.

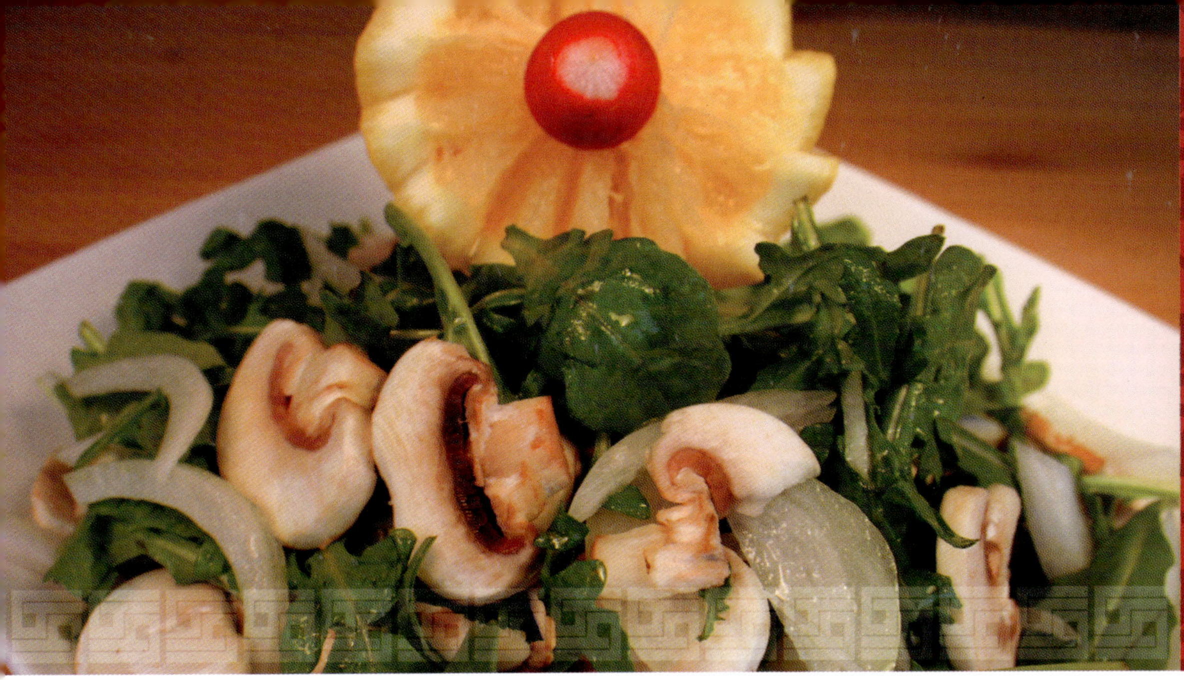

Arugula & Watercress Salad:

Salatet Rocca w'Jarjeer

سلطة روكا وجرجير

Ingredients

One 12-ounce bag arugula (rocca)
1 bunch watercress
½ teaspoon salt or to taste
1 small onion, sliced into thin wedges
2 tablespoons red vinegar
½ teaspoon crushed garlic
¼ cup extra virgin olive oil
1 cup sliced mushrooms

Start to Finish
10 minutes
Serves 6

Nutrition Information per Serving

Calories 93, Fat 9g, Saturated fat 1g, Cholesterol 0mg, Carbohydrate 3g, Fiber 0g, Protein 1g

Procedure

1• Wash arugula and watercress thoroughly and shake dry just before using, then place in a large bowl.

2• Sprinkle salt on the onion and mix well, then add to the bowl.

3• Mix vinegar, garlic and olive oil, pour it over the salad. Add mushrooms and fold to combine.

Serve it cold or at room temperature with any meal or as an appetizer.

** TIP Arugula is a rich source of iron, as well as of vitamins A and C. This salad tastes best when it is fresh.*

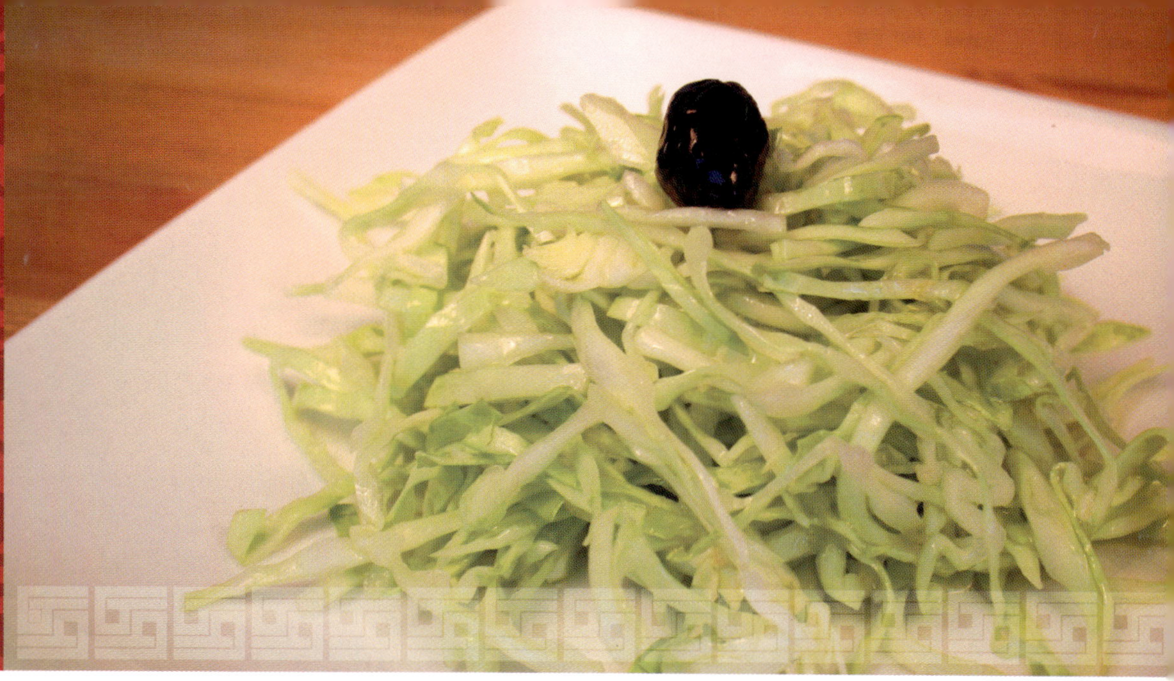

Cabbage Salad: Salatet Malfoof

سلطة ملفوف

Ingredients

4 cups very finely shredded cabbage
1 teaspoon fresh crushed garlic
½ teaspoon salt
¼ cup fresh lemon juice
¼ cup extra virgin olive oil

Start to Finish
7 minutes
Serves 4

Nutrition Information per Serving

Calories 140, Fat 14g, Saturated fat 2g, Cholesterol 0mg, Carbohydrate 5g, Fiber 2g, Protein 1g

Procedure

1• Place shredded cabbage in a large bowl.

2• In a small bowl, combine garlic, salt, lemon juice and oil.
Add to the cabbage, mix well to combine and serve.

Serve it cold or at room temperature with lamb kebabs or steak.

** TIP This salad may be prepared a day in advance and refrigerated in a covered container.*

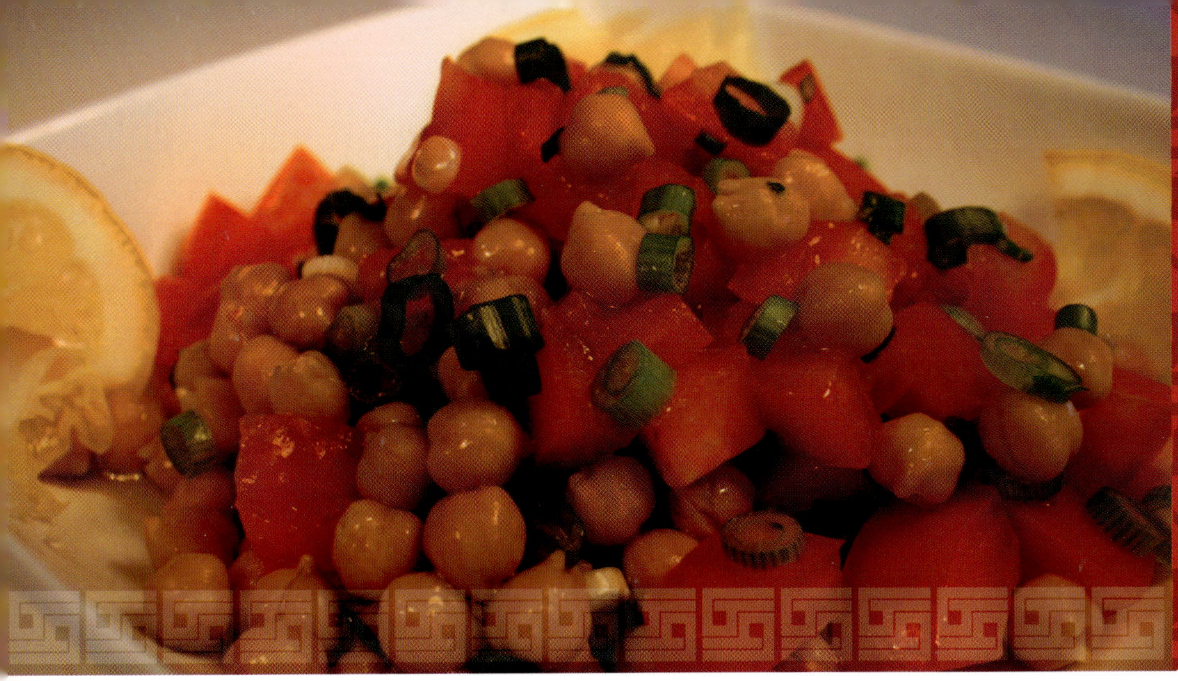

Chick-pea & Tomato Salad:

Salatet Hummus w'Banadourah

سلطة حمص وبندوره

Ingredients

3 cups Cooked Chick-peas
1 large tomato, diced into ¼-inch cubes (1cup)
½ cup thinly sliced scallions
2 cloves crushed garlic
½ teaspoon salt or to taste
¼ cup fresh lemon juice
¼ cup extra virgin olive oil

Start to Finish
10 minutes
Serves 4

Nutrition Information per Serving

Calories 469, Fat 15g, Saturated fat 2g, Cholesterol 0mg, Carbohydrate 66g, Fiber 19g, Protein 20g

Procedure

1• Put chick-peas, tomato, and scallions into a bowl and combine.

2• Mix garlic, salt, lemon juice and oil, add them to the chickpeas. Mix well and serve.

Serve it cold or at room temperature with fresh pita bread and radishes for breakfast, as a light lunch or dinner, or as an appetizer.

** TIP Chick-peas can be prepared a couple of days in advance.*

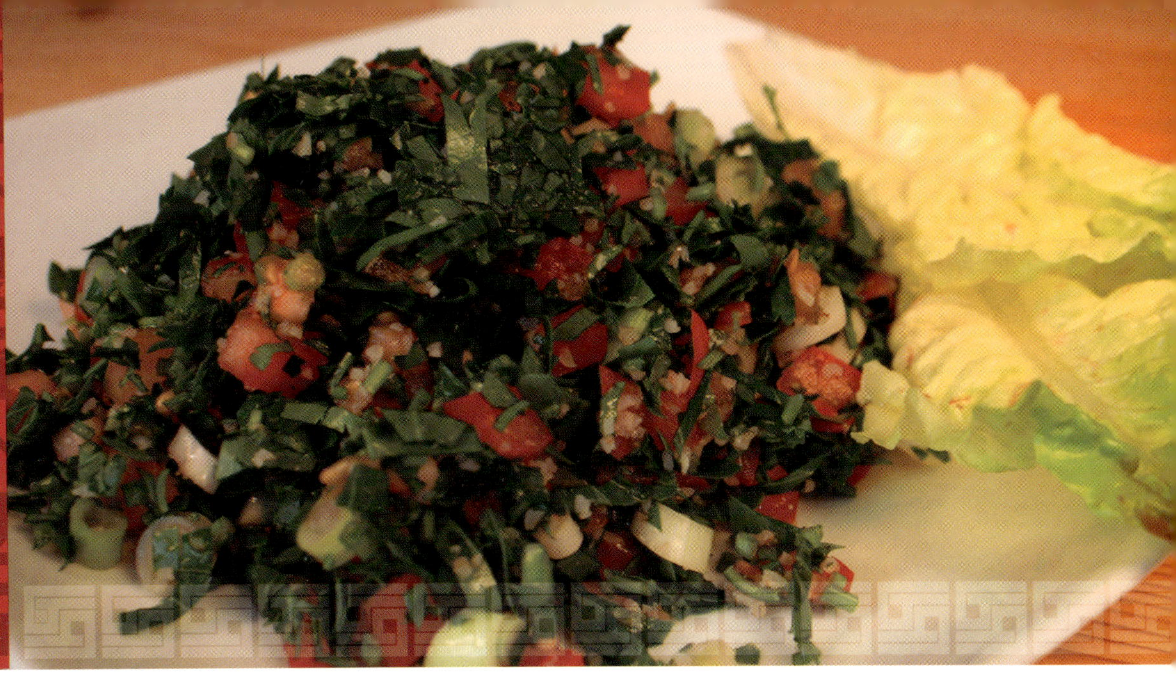

Fresh Produce with Crushed Wheat:

Tabbouleh

تبوله

Ingredients

2 tablespoons crushed wheat (burghul #1)
1 bunch or 2 packed cups of finely chopped parsley
¼ cup finely chopped mint leaves or 1 teaspoon dry mint
3 scallions, finely chopped
1 large tomato, finely diced
½ teaspoon salt or to taste
⅛ teaspoon ground black pepper
¼ cup lemon juice
2 tablespoons olive oil

Start to Finish
15 minutes
Serves 3

Nutrition Information per Serving

Calories 188, Fat 14g, Saturated fat 2g, Cholesterol 0mg, Carbohydrate 15g, Fiber 4.5g, Protein 3g

Procedure

1• Rinse cracked wheat 2 times in cold water, drain in a fine sifter and put in a medium-sized bowl.

2• Wash and drain parsley and mint, pat dry with a paper towel, then chop and add them to the cracked wheat.

3• Combine with chopped onion, diced tomato, salt, and pepper.

4• Pour in lemon juice and mix; add olive oil and mix again. Transfer to a platter & serve.

Serve it cold or at room temperature, with Romaine lettuce, white cabbage leaves, fresh tender grape leaves, or even with pita bread or chips. Whatever you choose will become your utensil as you use it to scoop up the Tabbouleh.

** TIP Tabbouleh tastes best when it is freshly combined, but vegetables can be prepared a day in advance if kept refrigerated separately in covered containers.*
Ingredients should be chopped only by hand.
Provides 36% of Vitamin A & 100% of Vitamin C daily requirements

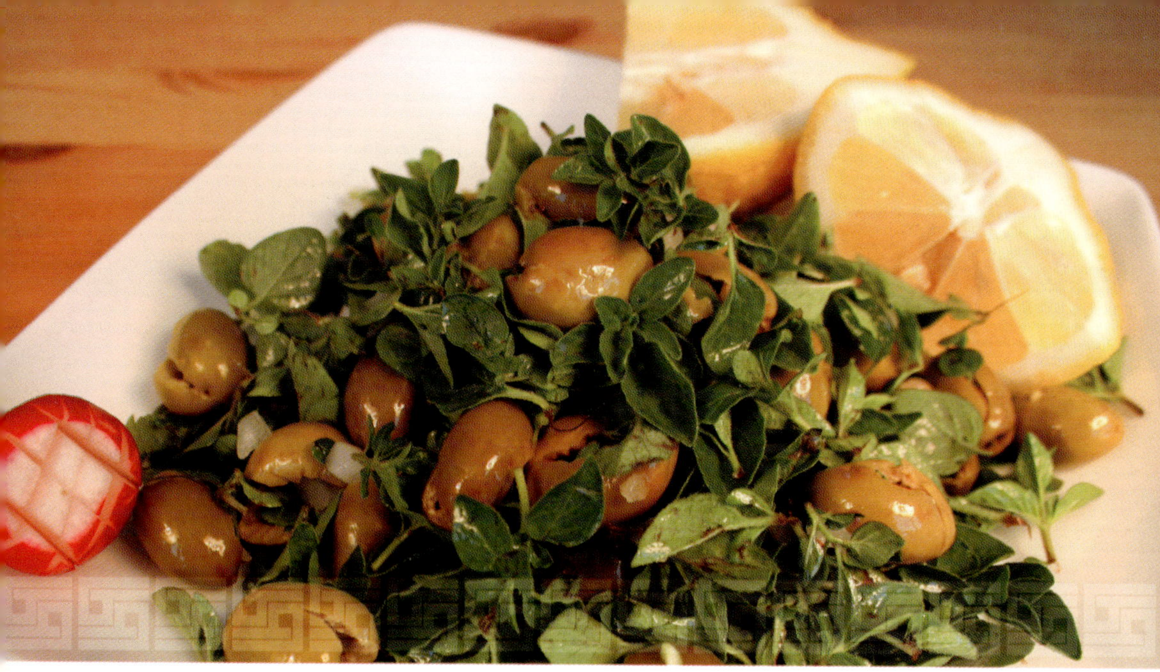

Fresh Oregano & Green Olives:

Salatet Zooba'a w'Zeitoon Akhdar

سلطه زوبع و زيتون اخضر

Ingredients

1 packed cup fresh oregano, washed and drained
½ cup pitted green olives
¼ cup finely sliced scallions
¼ teaspoon salt or to taste
2 tablespoons fresh lemon juice
2 tablespoons extra virgin olive oil

Start to Finish
7 minutes
Serves 4

Nutrition Information per Serving

Calories 95, Fat 10g, Saturated fat 1g, Cholesterol 0mg, Carbohydrate 2g, Fiber 0g, Protein 0g

Procedure

1• Combine all ingredients together and serve.

Serve it cold or at room temperature with bread as a salad or as an appetizer.

** TIP this dish may be prepared a couple of days in advance if stored in a covered container in the refregirator.*

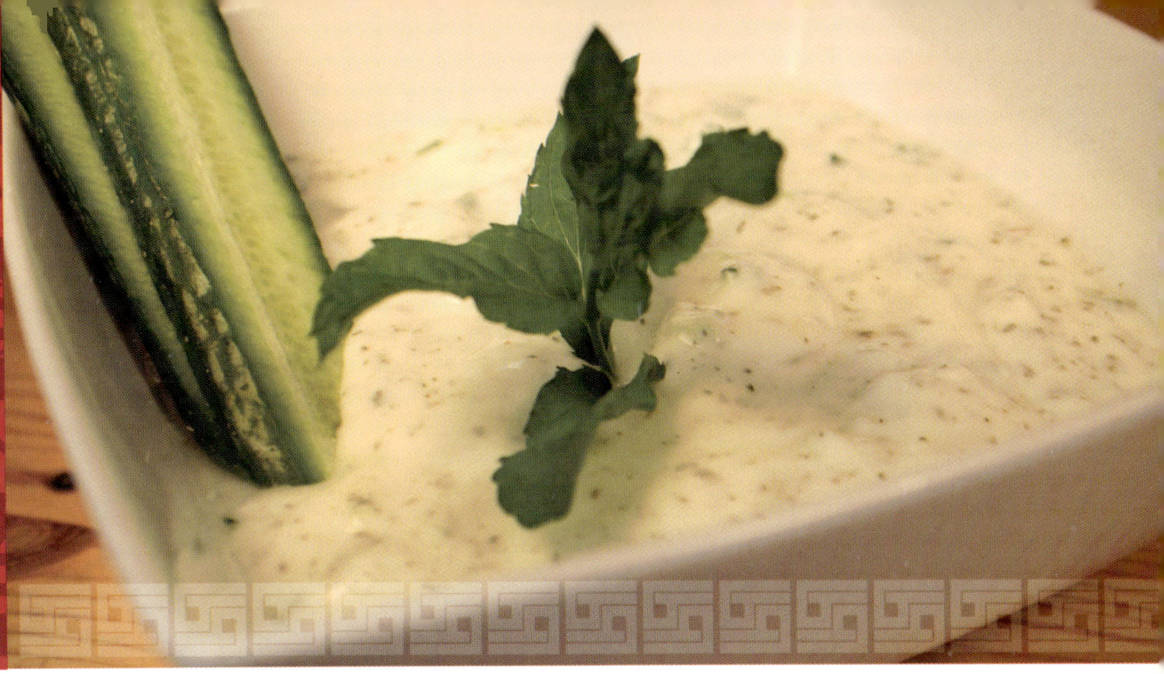

Yogurt Cucumber Salad: Laban bi Khyar

لبن بخيار

Ingredients

4 cups plain yogurt
6 small cucumbers peeled, quartered and thinly diced
2 medium garlic cloves, peeled and crushed
1 teaspoon salt or to taste
1 tablespoon dried mint, finely crushed, or to taste

Start to Finish
10 minutes
Serves 6

Nutrition Information per Serving

Calories 122, Fat 3g, Saturated fat 2g, Cholesterol 10mg, Carbohydrate 15.5g, Fiber 1g, Protein 9.5g

Procedure

1• In a large bowl, combine all ingredients and stir well.

Serve it cold or at room temperature as dip or salad with Kafta in Pita Bread, Baked Kibbeh or by itself as a light lunch.

** TIP salad can be prepared several days in advance if kept covered in the refrigerator.*

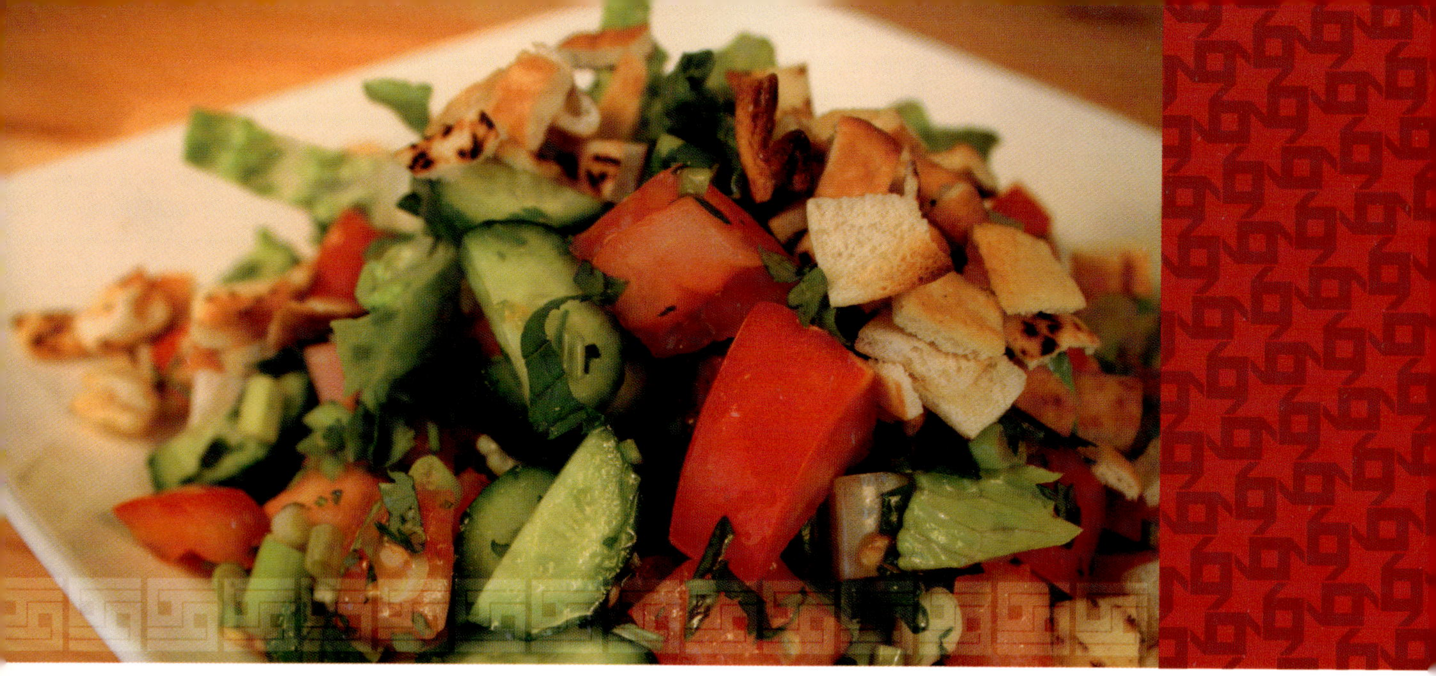

My family spent our summer vacations on the mountain of Hasroon, where most people grew a garden by the house. I clearly recall the crispy taste of a just-picked baby cucumber the size of my little finger. The produce vendors in the cities call these tiny cucumbers asabe'a el boubou ya khiar, meaning "the fingers of the baby."

I also have a vivid picture in my mind of street vendors pushing wooden carts loaded with fruits and vegetables near our city home, shouting funny verses about their wares and prices. I used to watch the neighbors as they bargained with the sellers from their balconies and as they rushed downstairs to pick up their vegetables. Others were clever enough to put money in a basket attached to a rope, and to throw it down to the vendor. The produce merchant caught the basket, removed the money, and replaced it with fruits and vegetables. Then the buyers pulled the basket back up to the balcony, saving themselves a trip down and back up the stairs.

Best of all was my mother's garden, which she grew on the balcony of our apartment building in the city. The balcony was filled with small pots of fragrant herbs and vegetables (Khodar الخضار) and she picked them fresh for the daily meal.

Salad with Toasted Bread: Fattoush

فتوش

Ingredients

1 loaf pita bread
1 cup tomato, diced
1 cup cucumber, diced
1 cup Romaine lettuce, finely chopped
½ cup thinly sliced scallions
⅓ cup chopped green pepper
½ cup finely chopped parsley
¼ cup chopped mint leaves
⅓ cup purslane leaves
½ teaspoon salt or to taste
1 teaspoon sumac

Dressing

¼ cup fresh lemon juice
1 teaspoon minced garlic
2 tablespoons extra virgin olive oil
Mix together and set aside.

Start to Finish
15 minutes
Serves 2

Procedure

1• Open pita bread, you will have 2 rounds. Toast, cool, and break into bite-sized pieces.

2• Mix dressing in a small bowl and set aside.

3• In a medium-sized bowl, combine remaining ingredients.

4• Pour dressing over the vegetable mixture and mix well.

5• Transfer mixture to a large platter and top it with the toasted bread. Serve immediately while the bread is still crunchy.

Serve it cold or at room temperature with Cracked Wheat with Lentils or by itself.

** TIP Fattoush can be prepared ahead of time by storing the dressing, bread and vegetables separately and combining them just prior to serving.*

Nutrition Information per Serving

Calories 244, Fat 14.5g, Saturated fat 2g, Cholesterol 0mg, Carbohydrate 27g, Fiber 4g, Protein 5g

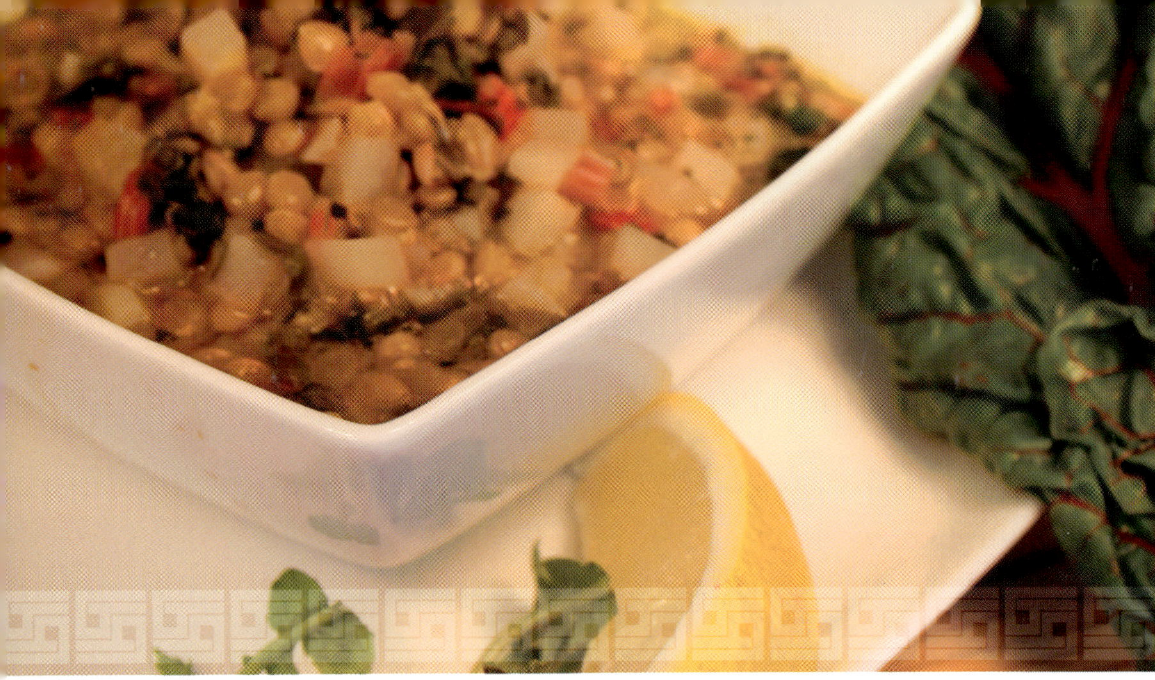

Lentils with Swiss Chard & Lemon Juice: Shorbit Adas b'Hamod

شوربة عدس بحامض

Ingredients

1 cup lentils, washed and drained
2 cups water
1 bunch Swiss chard, washed and finely chopped
1 medium potato, peeled and diced into ¼-inch cubes
4 cups hot water
¼ cup olive oil
1 medium onion, peeled and finely chopped
1 bunch cilantro, washed and finely chopped
1 tablespoon minced garlic
1 teaspoon salt
¼ teaspoon ground black pepper
2 tablespoons fresh lemon juice

Start to Finish
30 minutes
Serves 4

Procedure

1• Place washed lentils in a large pot with 2 cups water and bring to a boil over high heat. Cook over medium-high heat for 5 minutes.

2• Add chopped Swiss chard and chopped potato to the lentil pot. Pour in 4 cups hot water, stir, and bring to a boil for 10 minutes.

3• Put oil in a pan over medium heat, add chopped onion, and sauté until golden in color. Stir in chopped cilantro and minced garlic and cook for a minute, then turn off heat and add mixture to the lentil pot.

4• Sprinkle with salt and pepper, add lemon juice, stir, and simmer over low heat for 5 minutes.

Serve it hot or warm with radishes and toasted bread.

**TIP Lentils are rich in iron.*

Nutrition Information per Serving

Calories 333, Fat 10g, Saturated fat 1g, Cholesterol 0g, Carbohydrate 45g, Fiber 16g, Protein 18g

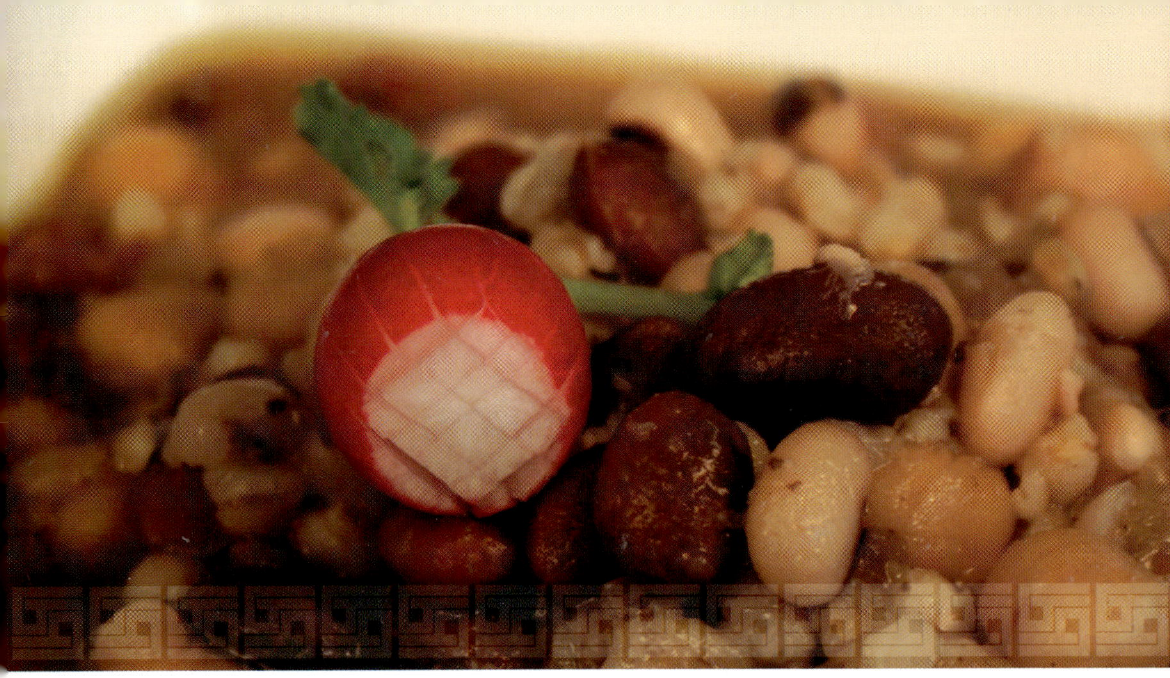

Mixed Grain Soup: Shorbit al Hooboob

شوربة الحبوب

Ingredients

¼ cup navy beans
¼ cup split broad beans
¼ cup pinto beans
¼ cup chick-peas
¼ cup black-eyed peas
¼ cup wheat

1 teaspoon salt or to taste
¼ teaspoon black pepper or to taste
¼ teaspoon seven spices
3 tablespoons olive oil
1 medium onion, chopped

Pressure pot

Start to Finish
30 minutes
Serves 6

Preparation

Sort and rinse beans in a colander under running water and soak overnight with 7 cups of water in the pressure pot.

Procedure

1• Place pot over high heat for 5 minutes, discard foam from the top, and stir. Cover according to pressure pot manual and cook for 20 minutes.

2• Meanwhile, put oil in a pan over medium-high heat, stir in onion, sauté until golden and set aside.

3• Open pressure pot following the manual instructions, add salt, pepper and seven spices, and stir well to combine. Stir in sautéed onion and oil, cook for a couple of minutes over medium heat, then serve.

Serve it hot or warm with radishes and fresh pita bread or Salad with Toasted Bread.

** TIP If you don't have a pressure pot, place grains in a heavy saucepan and cook covered for 1½ to 2 hours, or until beans are tender.*

Nutrition Information per Serving

Calories 230, Fat 9g, Saturated fat 1g, Cholesterol 0mg, Carbohydrate 29g, Fiber 8g, Protein 10g

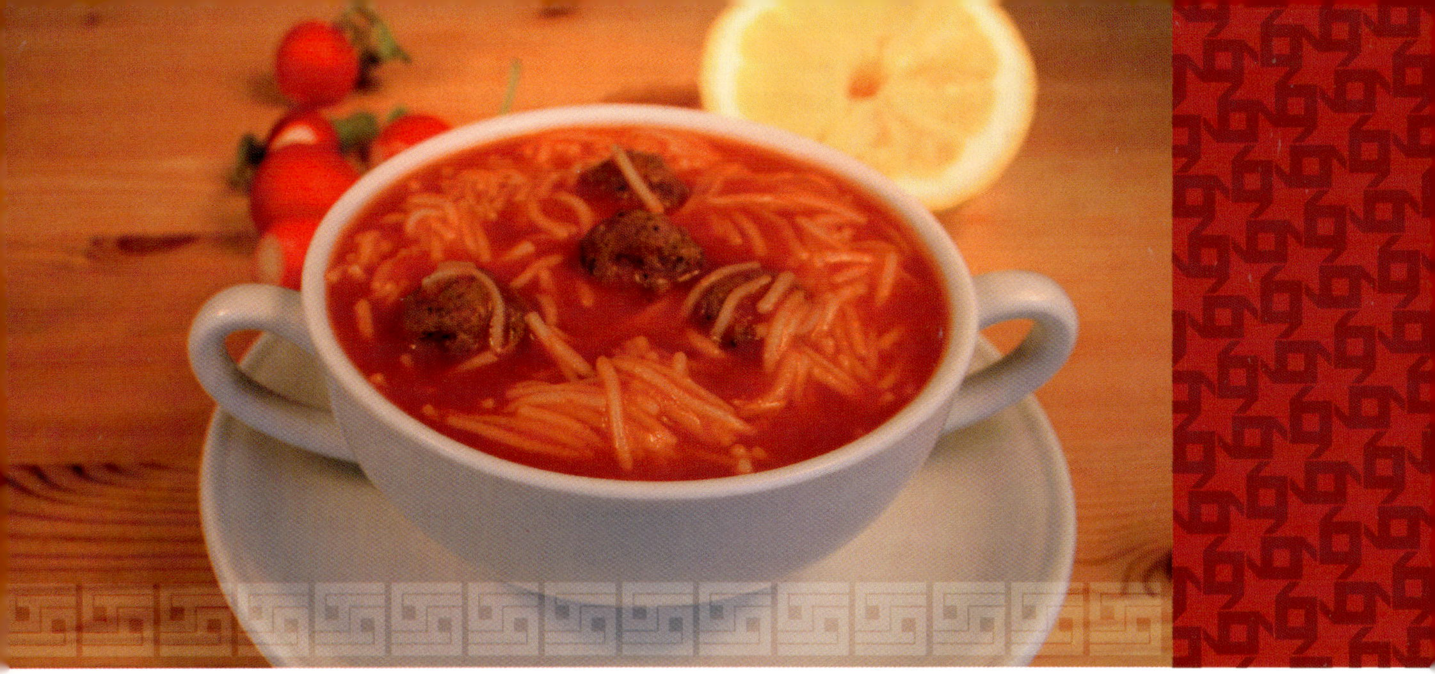

Vermicelli Soup: Shorbit al Sh'ayrieh

شوربة الشعيريه

Ingredients

1 pound ground lamb or beef
¼ teaspoon ground seven spices
¼ teaspoon cinnamon
¼ teaspoon ground black pepper
½ teaspoon salt or to taste

2 tablespoons clarified butter
2 tablespoons onion, very finely diced
1 cup vermicelli
2 cups tomato sauce
5 cups water
Salt and pepper to taste

Start to Finish
30 minutes
Serves 6

Procedure

1• Mix the first five ingredients together and form them into ¾-inch meatballs.

2• Place butter in a 2-quart pot over high heat, add onion and cook for 1 minute. Add meatballs and cook for 5 minutes or until nicely browned. Stir in vermicelli and cook for 1 more minute.

3• Add tomato sauce and water and bring to a boil for 2 minutes. Reduce heat to medium and cook for 7 minutes, turn off heat, and serve.

Serve it with French bread and salad.

***TIP The meatballs can be prepared a couple of days in advance if the meat is fresh.**

Nutrition Information per Serving

Calories 234, Fat 13g, Saturated fat 6g, Cholesterol 60mg, Carbohydrate 14g, Fiber 2g, Protein 16g

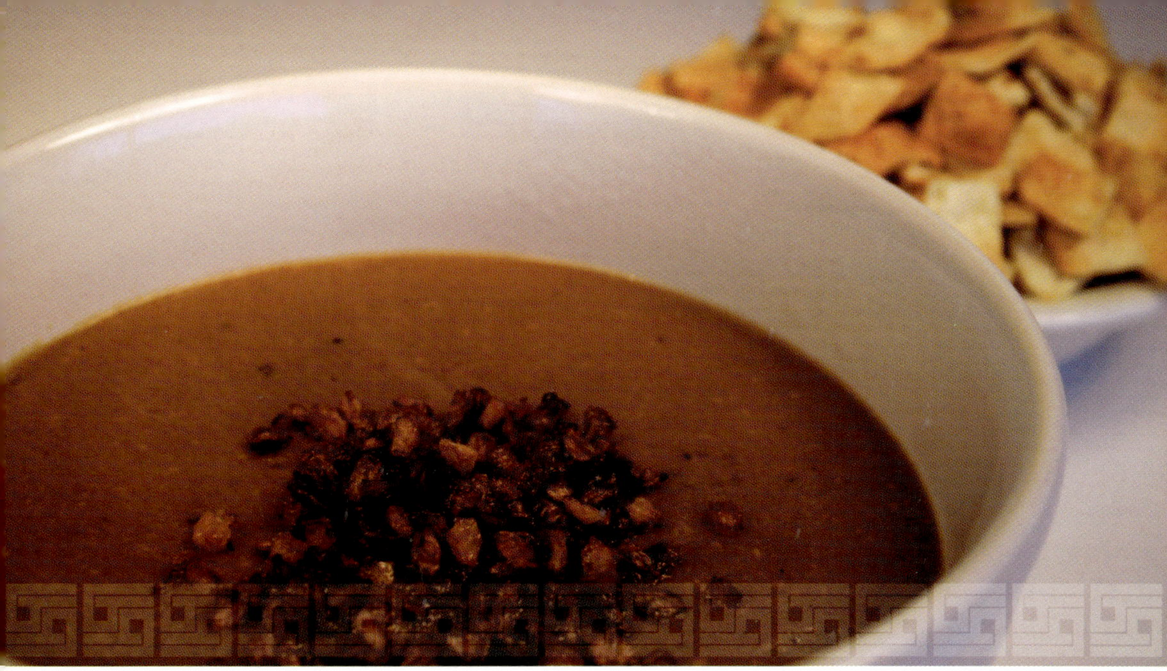

Lentil Soup: Shorbit al Adas

شوربة العدس

Ingredients

1 cup lentils, sorted, washed and drained
¼ cup rice, washed and drained
3 cups water
⅓ cup olive oil
1 medium onion, finely chopped
4 cups water
1 teaspoon salt or to taste
¼ teaspoon ground black pepper
Food processor or potato masher

Start to Finish
35 minutes
Serves 5

Nutrition Information per Serving

Calories 95, Fat 10g, Saturated fat 1g, Cholesterol 0mg, Carbohydrate 2g, Fiber 0g, Protein 0g

TOASTED PITA BREAD: 4 loaves pita bread , 2 tablespoons extra virgin olive oil Cut bread into ¾-inch squares using kitchen scissors, place in a pan, combine with oil and toast in heated oven until golden brown, stirring

Procedure

1• Pour 3 cups water into a large pot, stir in washed lentils and rice, and bring to a boil over high heat for 5 minutes. Reduce heat to medium, cover, and cook for 15 min.

2• Meanwhile, place oil in a medium pan over medium-high heat, stir in onions, and sauté until golden brown. Add cooked onions and hot oil to the lentil pot, stir, and turn off heat.

3• In a large saucepan, bring 4 cups water to a boil over high heat. Puree cooked lentils and rice in a food processor or mash with a potato masher.

4• While stirring, add lentil puree to the boiling water. Reduce heat to medium, add salt and pepper and cook for 10 minutes, stirring frequently. Turn off heat and serve.

Serve it hot or warm with Toasted Pita Bread and salad.

** TIP Leftover Toasted Pita Bread stays fresh in an airtight bag up to 2 months.*

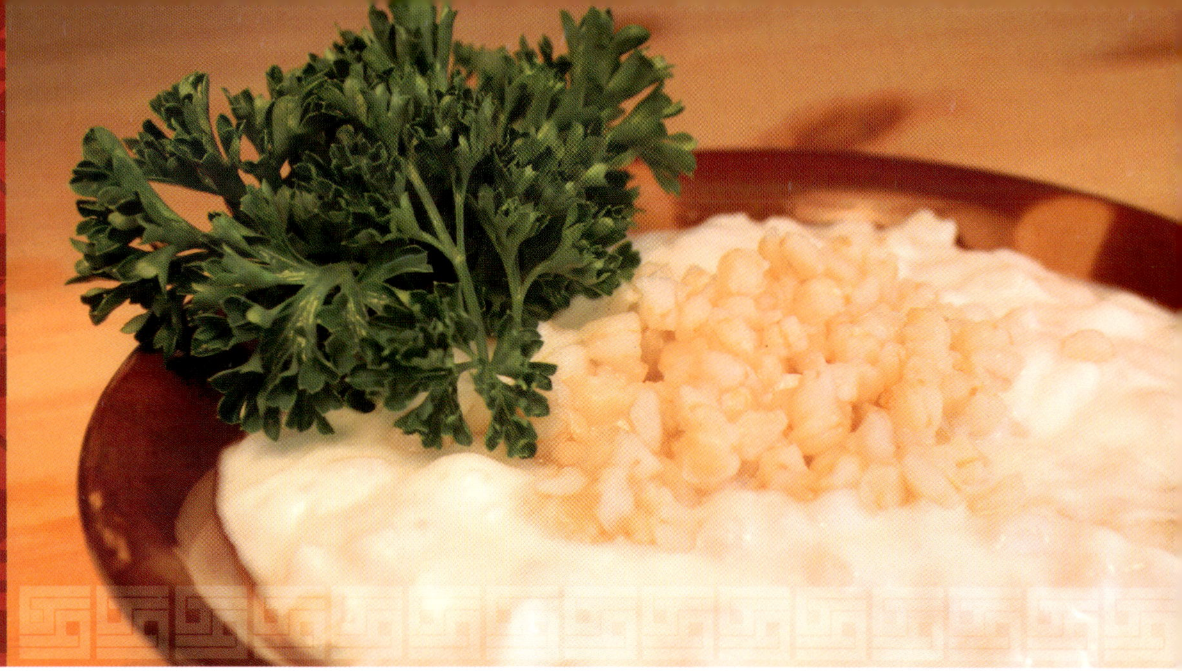

Yogurt with Wheat: Ameh b' Laban

قمح باللبن

Ingredients

1 cup whole grain wheat
4 cups water
4 cups plain yogurt
Salt to taste

Pressure pot

Start to Finish
30 minutes.
Serves 6

Nutrition Information per Serving

Calories 172, Fat 4g, Saturated fat 2g, Cholesterol 10mg, Carbohydrate 21g, Fiber 2.5g, Protein 13g

Procedure

1• Rinse wheat and place it with water in the pressure pot. Cover the pot and cook following the guidelines listed in your cooker instructions.

2• Drain cooked wheat, reserve liquid and let cool. Combine with yogurt and salt to taste. If you like it thinner, add some of the reserved liquid.

Serve it cold by itself as a light meal or snack.

** TIP This is an excellent light meal for the summer; it refrigerates well in a covered container for up to a week.*

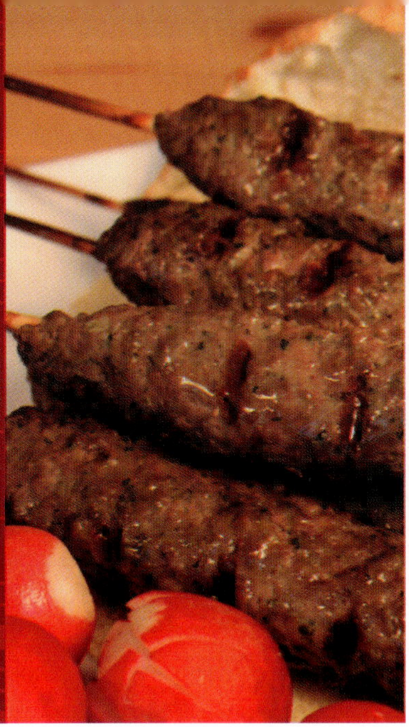
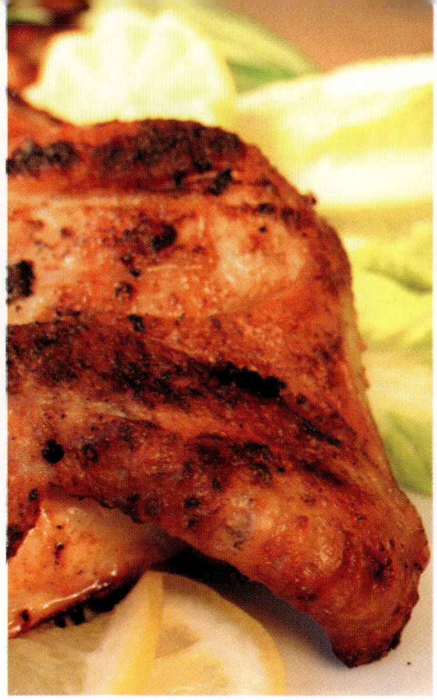
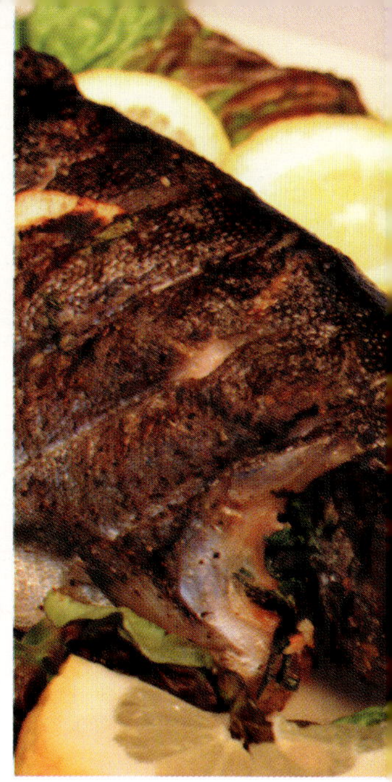

On the Grill: El Mashawi

المشاوي

The Lebanese love the out-of-doors, and they often spend their Sundays with family and friends in the mountains or near the beach. These occasions are perfect for a good meal of mashawi at a special dining spot. There is nothing like eating barbecued chicken with garlic dip at a mountain restaurant while gazing at a graceful waterfall or a panoramic view of the valley below. Most Lebanese live in apartment buildings, so the best place for them to barbecue their own meat, kafta (seasoned ground lamb), kebabs or seafood is on the balcony. This chapter is a favorite of my family with its variety of easy grilled entrees.

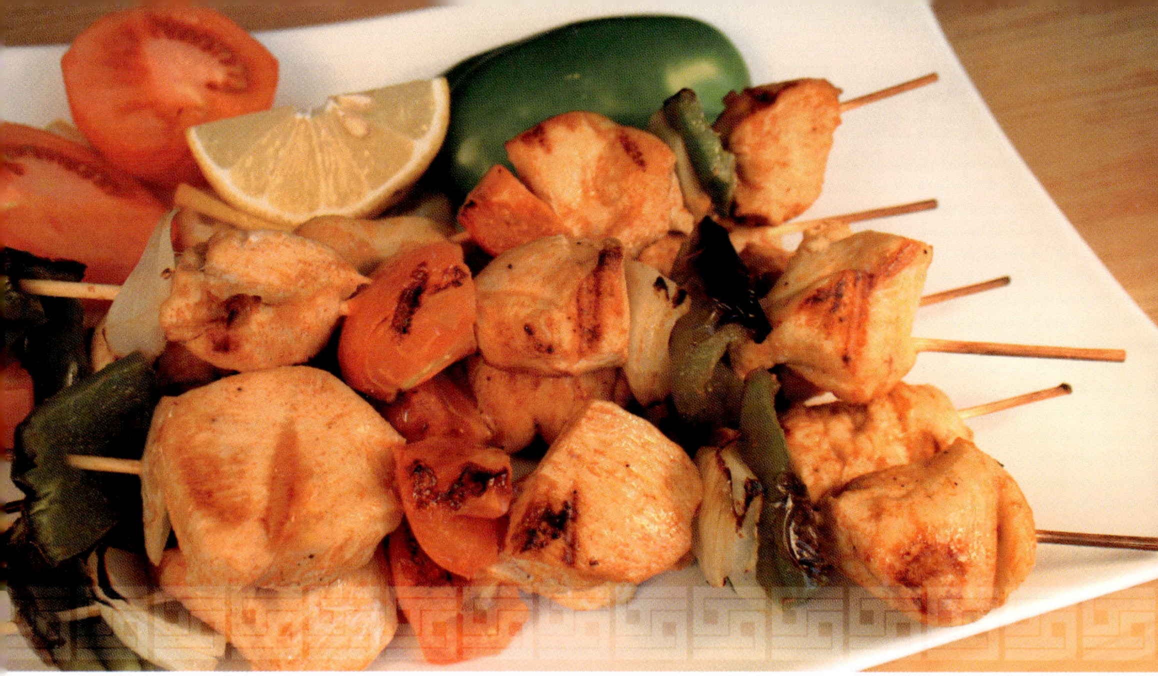

Chicken Kebabs: Shish Tawouk

شيش طاووق

Ingredients

1½ pounds chicken tenders
2 tablespoons fresh lemon juice
1 tablespoon crushed garlic
2 tablespoons olive oil
¼ teaspoon black pepper
¼ teaspoon paprika
½ teaspoon salt
4 small tomatoes, quartered
4 baby onions cut in half
1 green pepper, cut into eight 1½-inch wedges

8 wooden skewers soaked in water for 5 minutes

Start to Finish
30 minutes
Serves 4

Preparation: Garlic Sauce

- 7 Fresh cloves garlic, peeled and crushed
- 1 tablespoon fresh lemon juice
- ¼ cup extra virgin olive oil
- ½ teaspoon salt or to taste
- ½ cup mayonnaise

Food processor

Place all ingredient in the food processor, process well to fine texture and serve.

Procedure

1• Preheat grill on high (500 degrees F).

2• Rinse chicken, drain and pat dry with a paper towel. Cut each tender into 3 pieces and set aside.

3• On a deep platter, combine lemon juice, garlic, olive oil, black pepper, paprika and salt. Add chicken and cover completely with the marinade. Place tomato, onion, and green pepper on top and marinate for 7 minutes.

4• Place the chicken pieces onto the skewer. Alternate chicken with 2 tomato wedges and 1 piece of onion and pepper per skewer. Grill for 2 to 3 minutes on each side or until they are done.

Serve it hot with fresh pita bread, plain rice, Salad with Toasted Bread and Garlic Sauce.

** TIP Fresh chicken can be prepared on skewers a couple of days in advance if kept refrigerated in a covered container. If you feel too lazy to go outside to grill the chicken, just heat the oven to broil then place kebabs on the middle rack for 7 minutes on each side.*

Nutrition Information per Serving

Calories 403, Fat 18g, Saturated fat 4g, Cholesterol 122mg, Carbohydrate 13g, Fiber 3g, Protein 45g

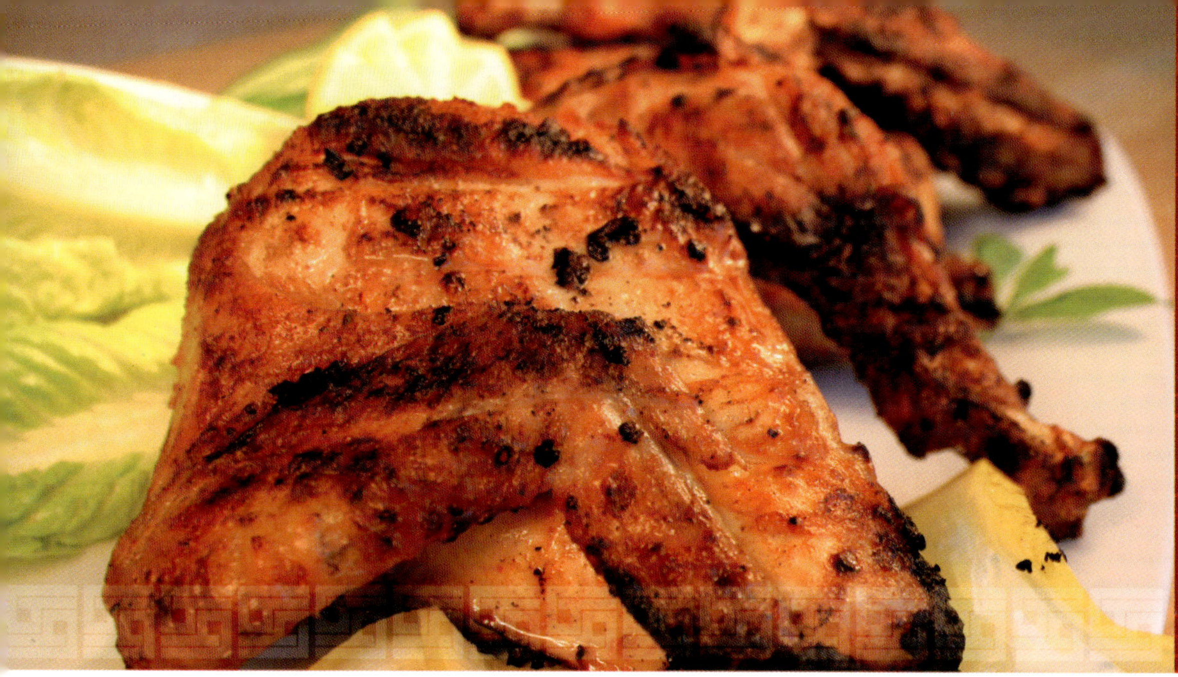

Grilled Chicken: Farouj Mashwi

فروج مشوي

Ingredients

1 small chicken
1 teaspoon salt or to taste
¼ teaspoon ground black pepper
¼ teaspoon paprika
2 tablespoons olive oil
2 tablespoons crushed garlic
¼ cup fresh lemon juice

Pastry brush
1 teaspoon crushed garlic
1 teaspoon fresh lemon juice
1 teaspoon oil
Fresh pita bread

Start to Finish
30 minutes
Serves 4

Procedure

1• Heat the grill on high (500 degrees F).

2• Rinse chicken with cold water, drain, and pat dry with a paper towel. Trim unnecessary fat, and cut into quarters.

3• Cut 2 slits on each of the thighs. Sprinkle chicken pieces with salt, black pepper and paprika, and rub the spices into the meat with your fingers. Mix oil, garlic and lemon juice, and pour it over the chicken pieces in a shallow baking pan. Marinate for 7 minutes.

4• Place chicken pieces on the hot grill. Discard the used marinade.

5• Combine 1 teaspoon each of crushed garlic, lemon juice and oil. Place in a small container by the grill for basting.

6• Grill chicken for 4 minutes on each side, then brush with the oil mixture and grill for 2 more minutes. Turn chicken over, brush again with oil and grill an additional 2 minutes. Continue this process until the chicken is done to your liking.

7• When chicken is cooked, place each piece inside a fresh pita bread to keep it moist.

Serve it hot or warm with hummus, Garlic Sauce and Salad with Toasted Bread.

** TIP Chicken can be marinated overnight if kept refrigerated in a closed container. Spread leftover Garlic Sauce on the inside of open pita bread and grill it. Yum!*

Nutrition Information per Serving

Calories 412, Fat 25g, Saturated fat 6g, Cholesterol 137mg, Carbohydrate 1g, Fiber 0g, Protein 42g

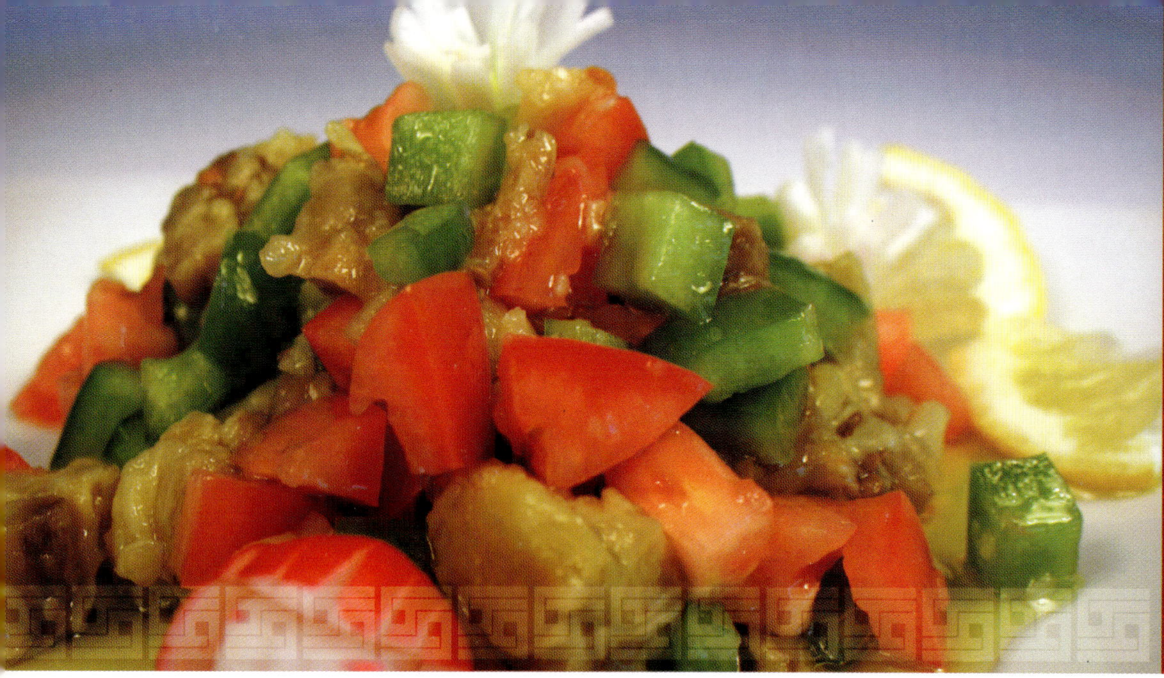

Grilled Eggplant: Bezenjaan Mashwi

باذنجان مشوي

Ingredients

2 large eggplants
1 green pepper, cut into ½-inch pieces
½ cup diced tomatoes

Start to Finish
20 minutes
Serves 6

Dressing

- 1 tablespoon crushed garlic
- 2 tablespoons fresh lemon juice
- ½ teaspoon salt or to taste
- ¼ cup extra virgin olive oil

Procedure

1• Preheat grill on high (500 degrees F).

2• Poke eggplants 3 times each with a knife and place on the grill. Turn them to cook evenly until they become soft. Remove from grill.

3• When cool enough to touch, hold each eggplant by the stem and peel under running cold water, then drain them in a colander. Discard the stem and burned peel.

4• Place eggplants on a large platter and either dice them with a knife or mash them with a fork. Prepare the dressing and mix well with the eggplant, then fold in chopped green pepper and diced tomatoes.

Serve it warm with fresh pita bread as an appetizer, or with grilled dishes.

** TIP Sprinkle grilled eggplants with salt to taste and 2 tablespoons fresh lemon juice and freeze up to a month for later use.*

Nutrition Information per Serving

Calories 132, Fat 9g, Saturated fat 1g, Cholesterol 0mg, Carbohydrate 13g, Fiber 7g, Protein 2g

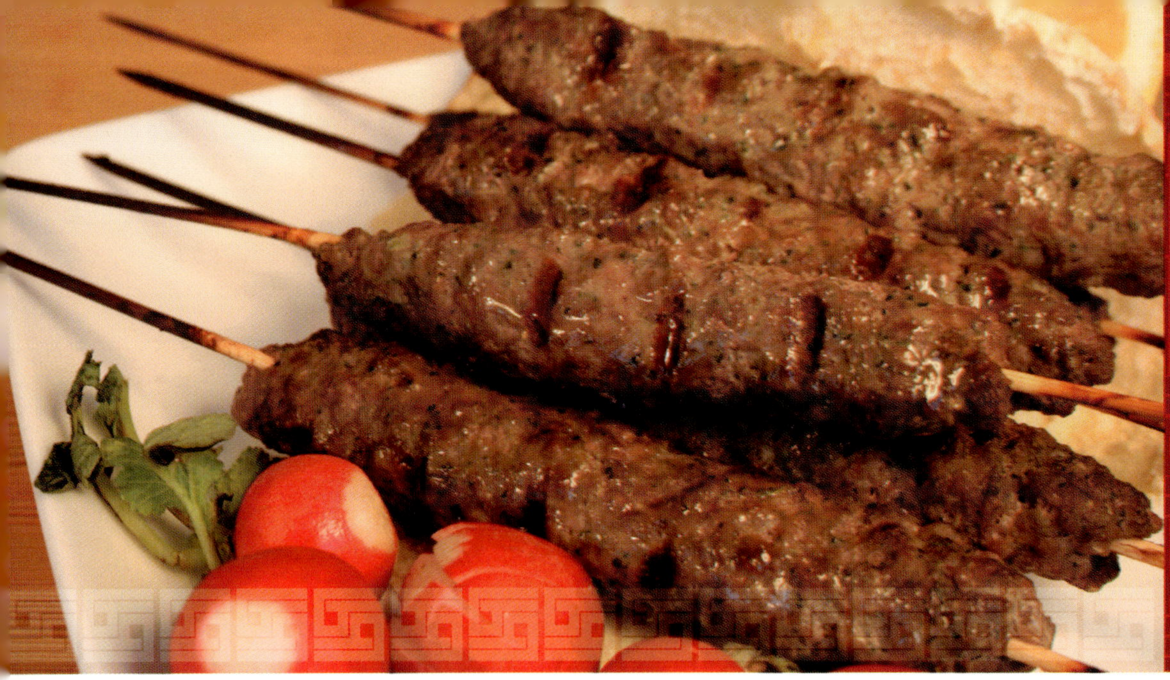

It is usually the butcher who prepares the traditional kafta in Lebanon. But in this recipe I will show you how to prepare your own by mixing ground meat, onion and parsley in an electrical food processor.

Kafta Kebabs: Kafta Mashwiyeh

كفته مشويه

Ingredients

One small bunch of parsley, washed, drained and chopped (1 cup packed)
1 medium onion, peeled and quartered
1 large clove garlic, peeled
1 pound extra lean ground lamb or beef
1 teaspoon salt
¼ teaspoon ground seven spices
¼ teaspoon ground black pepper
¼ teaspoon cinnamon
⅛ teaspoon crushed chili or to taste (optional)

Start to Finish
20 minutes
Serves 3

Electric food processor
6 skewers soaked in water for 5 minutes and set aside
3 fresh pita opened ¾ of the way along the side
½ teaspoon salt or to taste
¼ cup extra virgin olive oil

Procedure

1• Preheat the grill on high (500 degrees F) or start the barbecue.

2• Place parsley, onion, and garlic in the food processor. Pulse on and off until finely chopped, about 40 seconds.

3• Place ground meat in a large bowl and add salt, seven spices, black pepper, cinnamon, and crushed chili. Stir in the parsley mixture and blend well.

4• Divide the blended meat into 6 equal portions.

5• Wet your hands with cold water and roll one meat portion on a large cutting board with the palm of your hand into a 6- or 7-inch cylinder.
Finish the remaining meat portions in the same way and set aside.

6• Pierce each meat cylinder lengthwise through the middle with a skewer.
Grill evenly for 2 to 3 minutes or until cooked to your liking. (You can also grill them without the skewers).

7• Transfer the cooked meat cylinders from the skewers to the pita bread by placing 2 in each pita.

Serve it hot or warm with hummus or rice, Yogurt Cucumber Salad or Fresh Produce with Crushed Wheat.

** TIP If the meat is fresh you can prepare the meat skewers a day in advance and refrigerate in a covered container.*

Nutrition Information per Serving

Calories 292, Fat 17g, Saturated fat 7g, Cholesterol 100mg, Carbohydrate 3g, Fiber 0g, Protein 29g

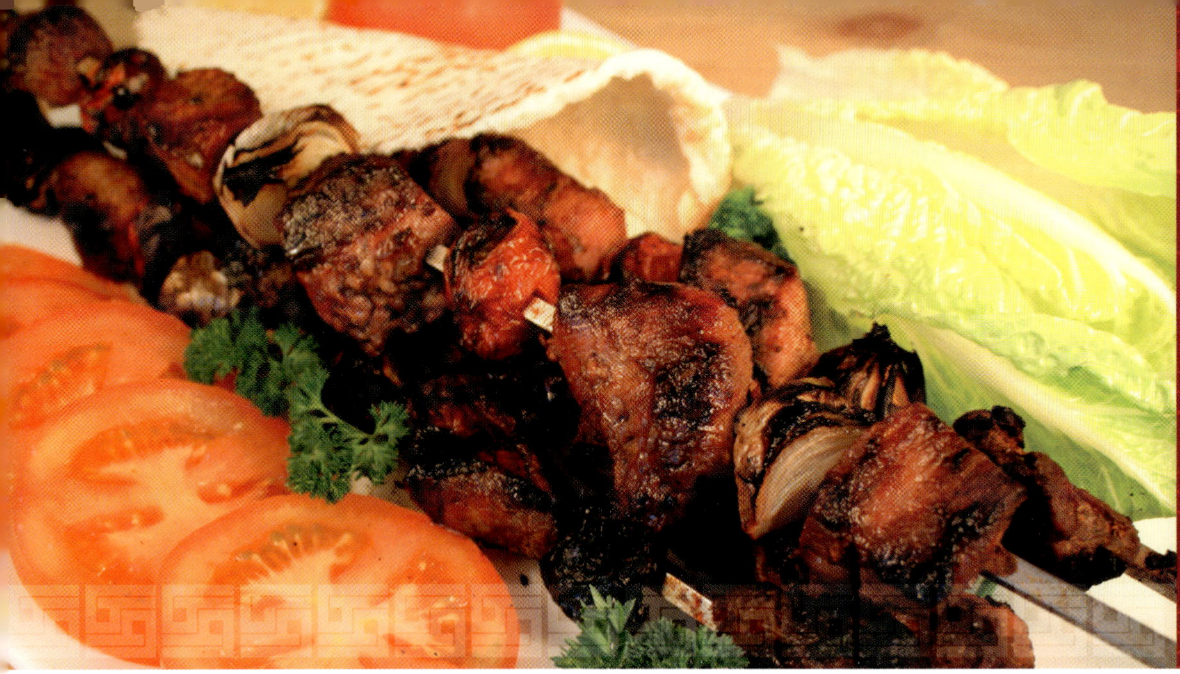

Lamb Kebabs: Shish Kebab

شيش كباب

Ingredients

1½ pounds extra lean lamb for grilling, cut into 1½-inch cubes
½ teaspoon salt
⅛ teaspoon ground black pepper
¼ teaspoon ground seven spices
⅛ teaspoon cinnamon
2 tablespoons minced garlic
2 tablespoons olive oil
8 baby onions, washed, patted dry and halved
16 baby tomatoes

8 wooden or metal skewers
2 fresh pita bread opened halfway along the seam

Start to Finish
25 minutes
Serves 4

Procedure

1• Heat the grill on high (500 degrees F).

2• In a large bowl, combine lamb pieces with salt, pepper, seven spices, cinnamon, garlic and oil. Mix well, then stir in onions and tomatoes. Marinate for 7 minutes.

3• Thread 5 pieces of meat onto each skewer, alternating with 2 pieces each of onion and tomato, leaving ⅛ of an inch in between each item.

4• Place the pita bread on a platter beside the grill.

5• Grill skewers about 2 minutes on each side. When the kebabs are almost done, remove them from the heat and place them on one open side of the bread. Flip the other side of the bread over the meat and press gently with your hand to soak up the juices from the meat, then remove the meat and return it to the grill.

6• When the kebabs are cooked to your liking, remove them from the grill and place them inside the bread to keep them moist and hot.

Serve it hot or warm with Garlic Sauce, fresh pita bread, hummus, and plain yogurt or Yogurt Drink.

** TIP Spread Garlic Sauce on the inside of open pita bread, then grill and enjoy.*

Nutrition Information per Serving

Calories 406, Fat 27g, Saturated fat 11g, Cholesterol 109mg, Carbohydrate 10g, Fiber 2g, Protein 29g

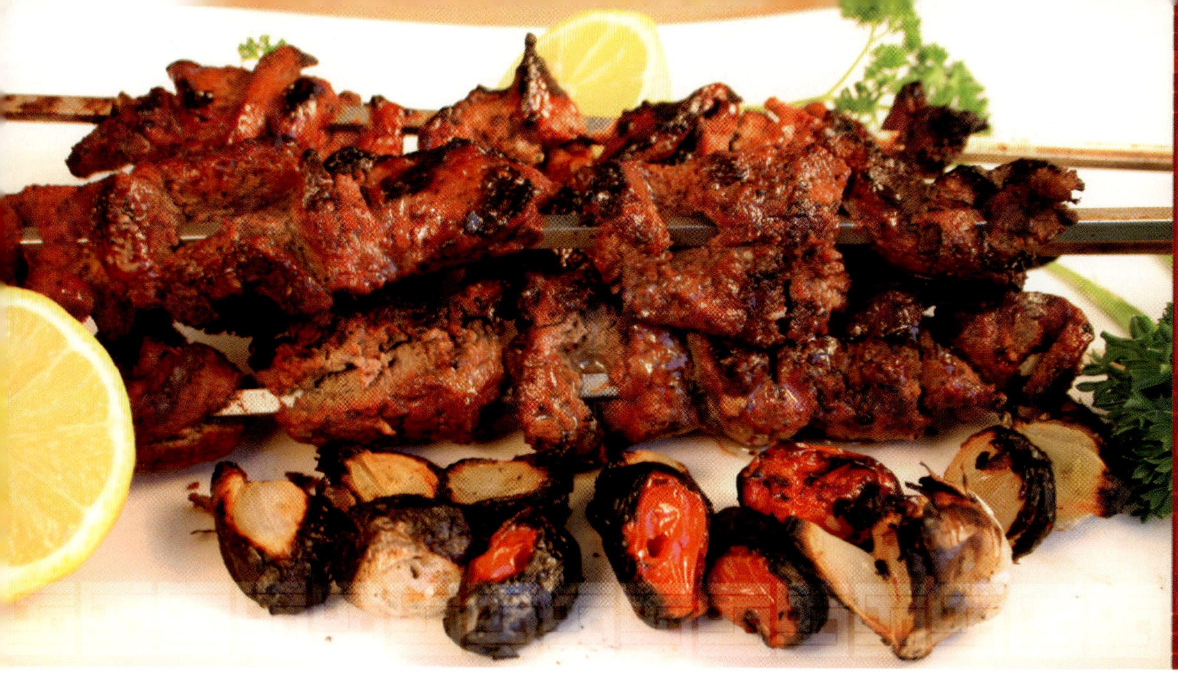

Liver Kebabs: Mila'k Mashwi

معلاق مشوي

Ingredients

1½ pounds lamb liver, cut into 1-inch cubes
½ teaspoon salt
1 teaspoon crushed garlic
¼ teaspoon ground black pepper
¼ teaspoon seven spices
⅛ teaspoon cinnamon
2 teaspoons vegetable oil

4 skewers soaked in water for 5 minutes
2 small fresh pita bread
Parsley and lemon wedges to garnish

Start to Finish
20 minutes
Serves 4

Procedure

1• Heat grill to high (500 degrees F).

2• Place liver cubes in a large bowl and coat with salt, garlic, pepper and seven spices. Pour in oil and mix well.

3• Thread liver pieces on the skewers, leaving ⅛ of an inch between each cube. Grill evenly, about 2 minutes on each side, or to your liking.

4• When kebabs are done, remove them from the grill and place them inside the pita bread to stay moist and hot.

Serve it hot by itself with pomegranate sauce, which can be purchased from any Middle Eastern store.

** TIP Liver can be prepared on skewers a day in advance if kept refrigerated in a closed container.*

Nutrition Information per Serving

Calories 175, Fat 8g, Saturated fat 2g, Cholesterol 358mg, Carbohydrate 4g, Fiber 0g, Protein 22g

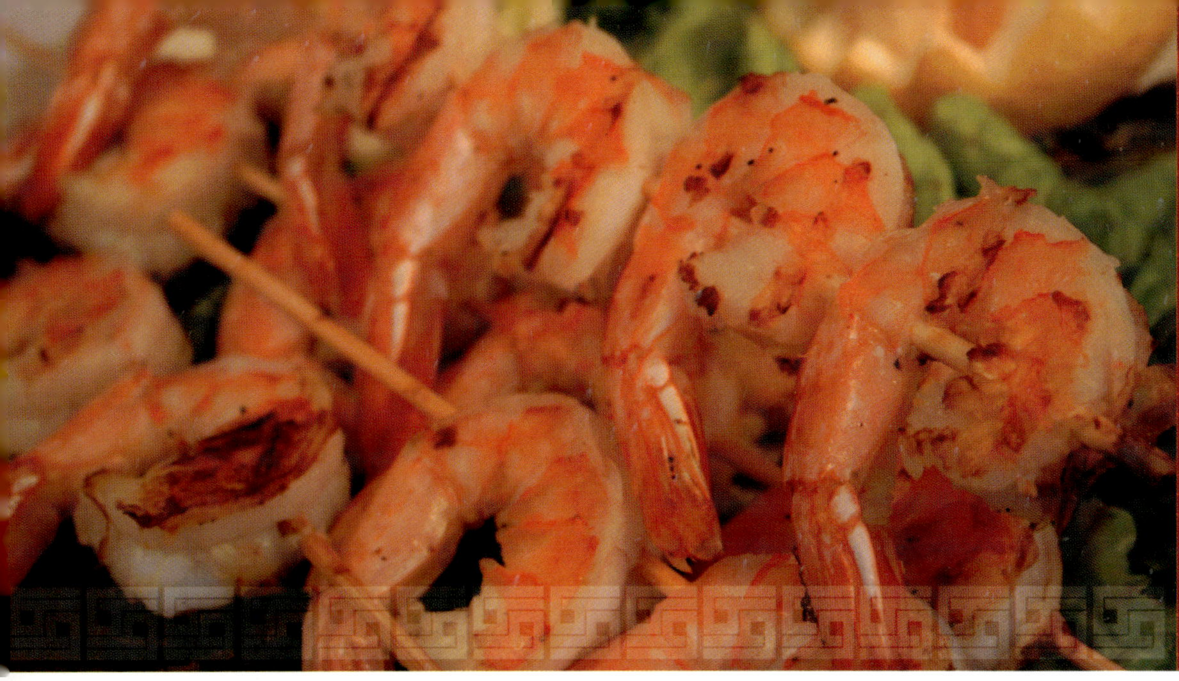

Shrimp Kebabs: Kraydes Mashwi

قريدس مشوي

Ingredients

1 pound large, raw shrimp, peeled and de-veined (about 16 shrimp)
2 tablespoons crushed garlic
1 teaspoon salt or to taste
¼ teaspoon ground black pepper
2 tablespoons olive oil

4 wooden skewers soaked in water for 5 minutes

Start to Finish
20 minutes
Serves 2

Procedure

1• Heat grill on high (500 degrees F).

2• Rinse shrimp and pat dry with a paper towel. Combine in a bowl with garlic, salt, pepper and olive oil. Marinate for 7 minutes.

3• Feed 4 shrimp onto each skewer, leaving ⅛ inch between each piece. Grill for 2 to 3 minutes or until shrimp are firm and pink.

Serve it hot or warm with baked potato and hummus or Salad with Toasted Bread.

** TIP Fresh shrimp can be prepared a few days in advance if kept refrigerated in a covered container.*

Nutrition Information per Serving

Calories 138, Fat 9g, Saturated fat 2g, Cholesterol 88mg, Carbohydrate 1g, Fiber 0g, Protein 12g

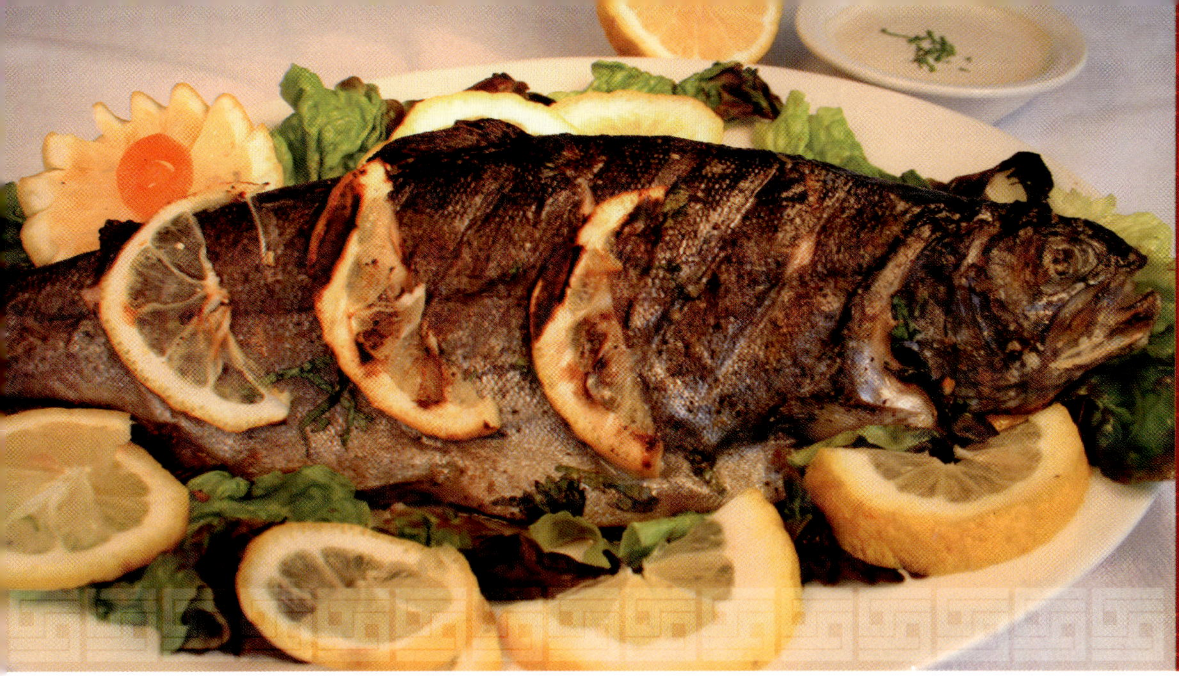

Whole Grilled Trout: Samakeh Mashwiyeh

سمكه مشويه

Ingredients

1 fresh, large, whole trout (about 2 pounds)
1 teaspoon salt
¼ teaspoon ground black pepper
¼ teaspoon seven spices
2 tablespoons olive oil
1 small bunch cilantro, washed and finely chopped, or 1 cup packed
2 tablespoons crushed garlic

Lemon wedges, thinly sliced
1 slotted aluminum foil sheet

Start to Finish
25 minutes
Serves 4

Procedure

1• Heat grill to high (500 degrees F).

2• Rinse fish and pat it dry with a paper towel. Combine salt, pepper and spices. Sprinkle mixture both on the surface and inside the trout, and rub it in with your fingers. Pour oil onto the fish and rub it all over the skin as well.

3• Combine cilantro and garlic, and stuff half of it into the mouth of the trout. Make 2 slits in the middle of the fish and fill them with the remaining cilantro mixture. Place 3 lemon wedges on the stuffed trout and marinate for 7 minutes.

4• Put slotted foil sheet on a heated grill and line the middle of it with 3 lemon wedges. Place trout over the lemon and grill for 4 minutes on each side or until done.

5• Remove trout from foil sheet to a platter and serve.

Serve it hot or warm with tahini sauce (tarator), Salad with Toasted Bread, or baked potato and Salad.

** TIP Fresh trout can be marinated overnight if kept refrigerated in a closed container. For a delicious, one-stop meal, try grilling fresh corn, asparagus, sliced eggplant and scallions with the trout.*

Nutrition Information per Serving

Calories 187, Fat 11g, Saturated fat 2g, Cholesterol 56mg, Carbohydrate 1g, Fiber 0g, Protein 20g

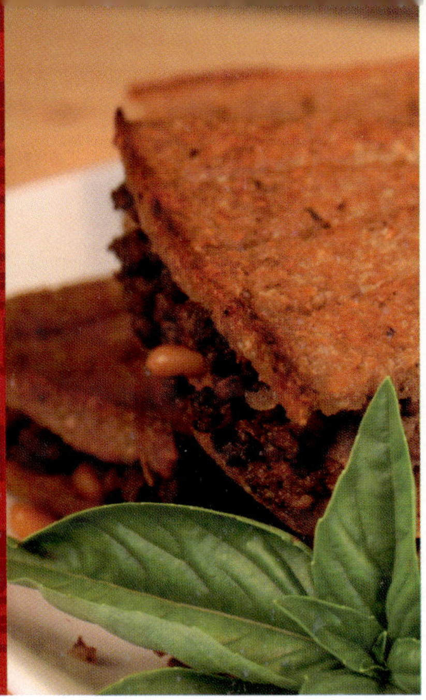 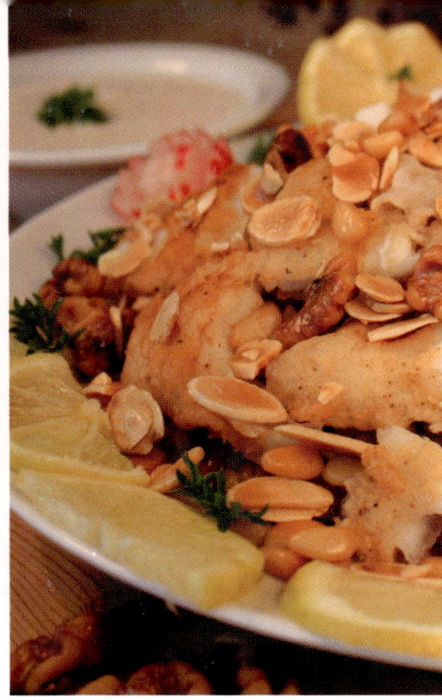 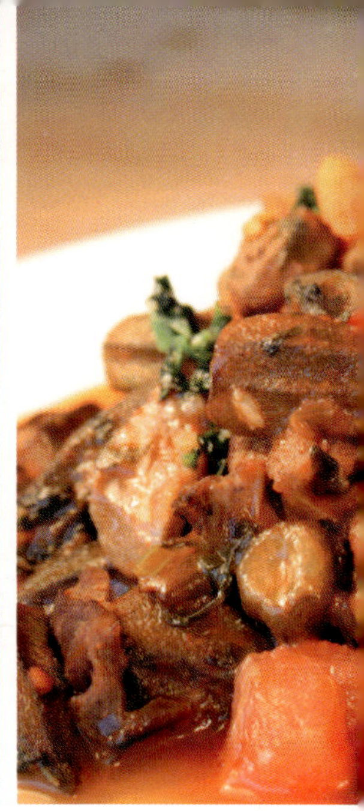

Main course: El Sahin El Ra'eecy

الصحن الرئيس

Lebanese dishes are made up of a variety of great tastes. Meats, cracked wheat, grains, legumes and vegetables make up a large part of the diet. Lamb is a favorite, along with red mullet and chicken.

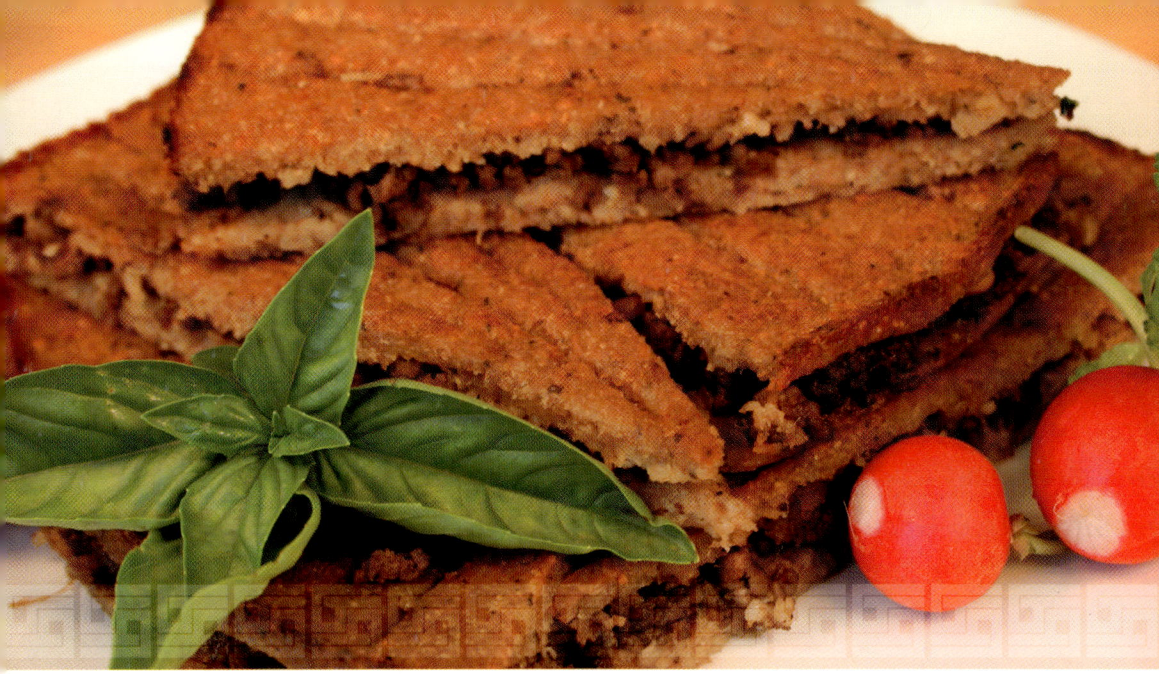

Kibbeh كبه *is a national dish, one of Lebanon's most appetizing and versatile staple foods. It can be eaten as part of the Mezze (Lebanon's traditional hors d'oeuvres), as a buffet finger-food or as a main course at lunch or dinner. The basic mixture of pounded meat, onion and herbs, combined with salt, spices and fine cracked wheat (or burghul #1), gives it a special texture and taste. I clearly remember my mother pounding the meat mixture in a mortar and pestle until it turned into a smooth paste. Luckily, we now have food processors -- no need to pound anymore!*

Baked kibbeh (kibbeh bil saniyeh) is an oven-baked main course dish. It consists of a layer of meat filling (hashweh) between top and bottom layers of kibbeh. The Lebanese enjoy many kinds of kibbeh. The Zgharta, Ehden, Beshari and Hasroon mountains are well known for serving good raw kibbeh (kibbeh nayeh) and grilled kibbeh (kibbeh mashwiyeh).

Baked Kibbeh: Kibbeh bil Saniyeh

كبه بالصينيه

Ingredients

1 recipe Kibbeh Dough
1 recipe Meat with Pine Nuts
1 foot x 3 feet of plastic wrap
Rolling pin
Greased 9 x 11 x 1½-inch pan
⅓ cup clarified butter

Preparation

- Kibbeh Dough prepared and set aside.
- Meat with Pine Nuts prepared and set aside.

Start to Finish
30 minutes
plus prepared recipes and baking
Serves 6

Procedure

1• Preheat oven to 400 degrees F.

2• Split the dough into two equal parts.

3• Spread plastic wrap on working surface. Dip your fingers in ice cold water and wet half of the plastic wrap with your fingers so the dough will not stick. Place one part of kibbeh dough in the middle of the wet plastic wrap. Press it flat to make a rectangle.

4• Wet fingers again and run them over the dough, then fold the plastic wrap over the wet dough. Roll the plastic-covered dough with a rolling pin until it is ¼ inch in thickness or less.

5• Place the pan lightly over the covered dough to make sure that the dough will cover the entire bottom of the pan. Set the pan aside.

6• Gently uncover the top plastic wrap. Carefully invert the dough and place it into the greased pan so that the raw dough is at the bottom of the greased pan and the plastic wrap covers the top of the dough.

7• Pull off remaining wrap and reserve it for the second part of the dough.

8• Dip your hand in the ice water and pat the dough gently to insure that it is spread evenly to the edges of the pan. This is the bottom layer of the kibbeh.

9• Spread meat filling to cover the dough in the pan and set aside.

10• Roll out the second piece of dough in the same manner as the first. Invert rolled dough over the meat filling to cover it. Gently remove the plastic wrap and discard.

11• Wet your fingers with ice water and lightly smooth the top layer so that it touches the sides of the pan.

12• Spread ⅓ cup clarified butter on top. With a knife, mark the top layer of kibbeh into diamond shapes. Bake kibbeh for 30 minutes on second oven rack.

Serve it hot or warm with plain yogurt, Baba Ghanouj, fresh radishes or Salad.

** TIP Kibbeh dough can be made into a patty and fried, then topped with a filling or eaten plain. Kibbeh freeze well for up to 2 months.*

Nutrition Information per Serving

Calories 348, Fat 20g, Saturated fat 7g, Cholesterol 81mg, Carbohydrate 2g, Fiber 3g, Protein 26g

Kibbeh Dough: Ajeenet el Kibbeh

عجينه الكبه

Ingredients

2 cups fine cracked wheat (burghul #1)
1 pound extra lean, very finely-ground lamb or beef
1 medium onion
1 teaspoon salt
¼ teaspoon ground seven spices
¼ teaspoon ground white pepper
¼ teaspoon ground cinnamon
2 tablespoons finely-chopped fresh mint or basil leaves

Electric food processor
1 cup water
1 cup ice cubes

Start to Finish
10 minutes

Procedure

1• In a large bowl, wash burghul with cold water several times, drain well and set aside.

2• Grate onion over the burghul with a fine hand grater. Add ground meat. Sprinkle with salt, seven spices, black pepper, and ground cinnamon, and mix to form meat dough.

3• Split both meat dough and chopped mint into three equal parts. Place one part of the dough in the food processor. Add one part chopped mint, one tablespoon water and one ice cube. Process until dough sticks together and forms a ball, about 40 seconds.

4• Remove kibbeh dough from processor and finish the remaining two parts of the meat dough in the same way.

5• Combine all the kibbeh dough with your hands in a large bowl and set aside until needed.

** TIP The dough should be manageable and soft.*

Nutrition Information per Serving

Calories 180, Fat 8g, Saturated fat 3g, Cholesterol 54mg, Carbohydrate 14g, Fiber 3g, Protein 12g

Meat with Pine Nuts:

Hashwet Lahmeh w'Snoubar

حشوه لحمه وصنوبر

Ingredients

1 tablespoon vegetable oil
⅓ cup pine nuts
1 pound extra lean beef or lamb
½ teaspoon salt or to taste
¼ teaspoon ground seven spices
¼ teaspoon ground black pepper
¼ teaspoon ground cinnamon

Start to Finish
15 minutes

Procedure

1• Sauté pine nuts in oil over medium-high heat until golden brown (careful, they burn easily). Transfer nuts with a slotted spoon to a platter lined with paper towels. Reserve oil.

2• Add meat to the reserved oil and cook over medium-high heat until meat is brown and juice evaporates, about 5 minutes.

3• Sprinkle meat with salt, seven spices, black pepper and cinnamon; stir well and turn off heat. Add toasted pine nuts and set aside.

** TIP This filling can be prepared a few days in advance. It is a delicious topping for Lebanese Spaghetti. Pine nuts also can be toasted in a hot oven for a couple of minutes while the meat is cooking.*

Nutrition Information per Serving

Calories 135, Fat 10g, Saturated fat 3g, Cholesterol 33mg, Carbohydrate 1g, Fiber 0g, Protein 11g

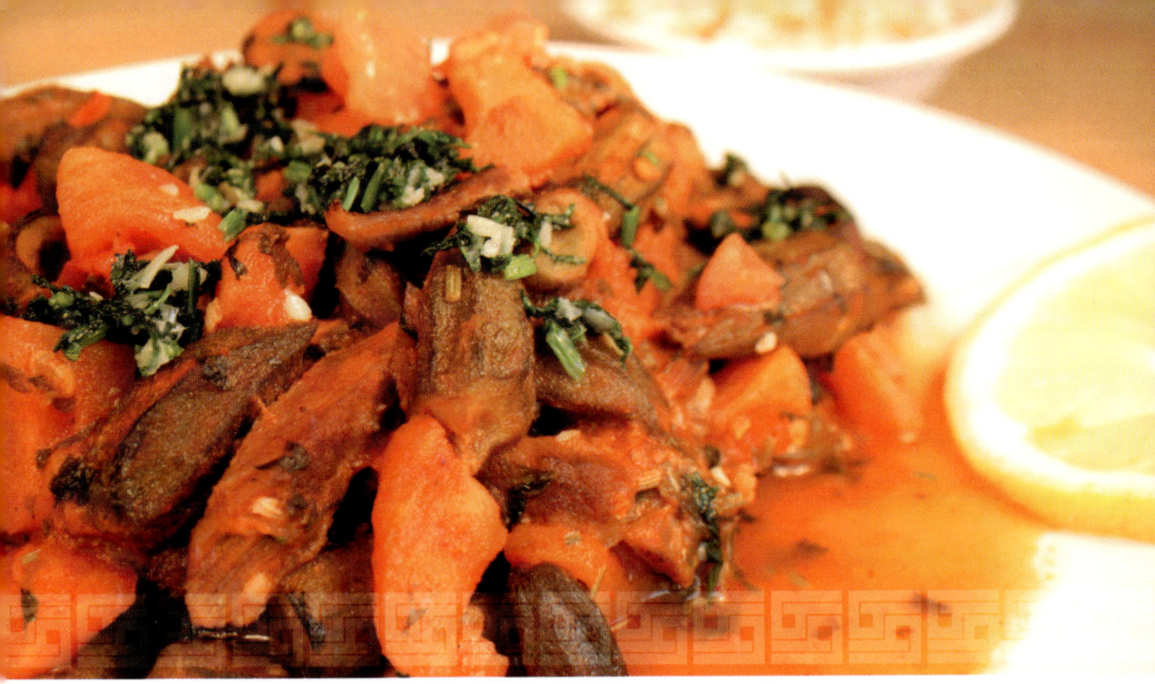

Baby Okra with Tomato and Garlic:

Bamyeh b'Zeit

بامیه بزیت

Ingredients

1 pound frozen baby okra, thawed
2 tablespoons vegetable oil
½ teaspoon salt

3 tablespoons olive oil
1 large onion, cut into 1-inch cubes
½ cup peeled whole garlic
2 cups tomatoes, peeled and diced
2 tablespoons lemon juice
15 oz can of chick-peas, rinsed and drained
1 cup chopped cilantro
¼ teaspoon ground black pepper
1 teaspoon salt
1 cup water

Large pan

Start to Finish
30 minutes
plus prepared
recipes and baking
Serves 6

Preparation

• Heat oven to 450 degrees F.
• Strain okra and pat dry with paper towel.
• Put 2 tablespoons oil in a large pan, add okra, sprinkle with salt and mix well. Place in the oven to cook for 15 minutes or until golden brown, stirring frequently. Set aside when done.

Procedure

1• Meanwhile, pour 3 tablespoons olive oil in a skillet over medium-high heat, add onion and garlic, and sauté for 3 minutes. Add tomatoes and lemon juice, stir, and cook for several more minutes.

2• Stir in chick-peas and cilantro and cook covered for 5 minutes.

3• Uncover the skillet and add cooked okra, pepper, salt, and 1 cup water. Stir and bring to a boil, then reduce heat to medium and stir again. Cook for 10 more minutes; remove from heat and set aside, ready to serve.

Serve it hot, warm or cold with salad and pita bread or rice, or as an appetizer.

***TIP Okra can be prepared a couple of days in advance.**

Nutrition Information per Serving

Calories 373, Fat 20g, Saturated fat 2g, Cholesterol 0mg, Carbohydrate 43g, Fiber 11g, Protein 11g

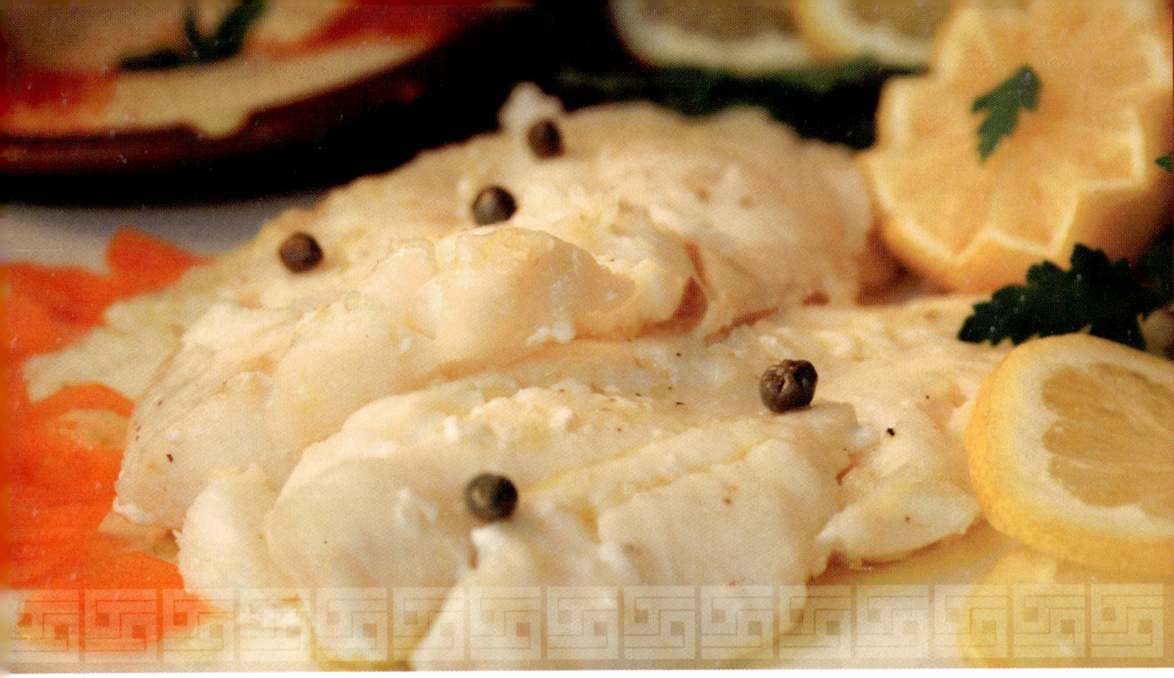

Baked Fish Fillets in Garlic Sauce:

Samak b'Zeit w'Toom

سمك هبره مشوي بالفرن

Ingredients

2 pounds orange roughy fillet
½ teaspoon salt or to taste
2 tablespoons crushed garlic
¼ cup olive oil
¼ teaspoon ground black pepper
¼ teaspoon seven spices

Medium pan
Pastry brush

To garnish

- lemon wedges and parsley sprigs

Start to Finish
25 minutes
Serves 4

Procedure

1• Heat oven to 450 degrees F.

2• Wash fish, drain, and pat dry with a paper towel, then sprinkle salt all over it.

3• Combine garlic with olive oil in the pan and place fish fillets in it. Sprinkle pepper and seven spices, and then brush the fish with the garlic-olive oil from the pan.

4• Bake for 10 minutes, remove pan from oven and turn over the fish. Place it back in the oven to bake for another 10 minutes.

5• Serve on a platter garnished with lemon wedges, parsley and capers.

Serve it hot or warm with baked potatoes, hummus, and a salad of your choice.

** TIP To eliminate the smell of fish, soak fillets in ice water and salt for a few minutes and drain before using.*

Nutrition Information per Serving

Calories 275, Fat 15g, Saturated fat 2g, Cholesterol 44mg, Carbohydrate 1g, Fiber 0g, Protein 32g

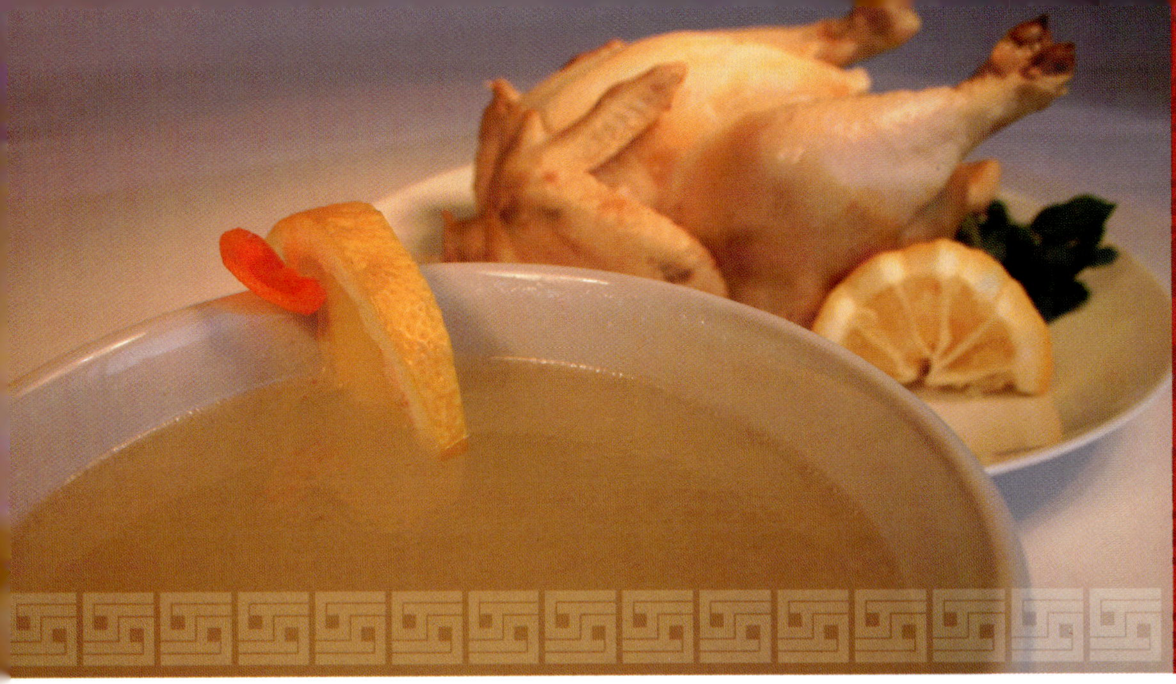

Chicken Broth: Makr'it Dajaj

مرقة دجاج

Ingredients

2- to 3-pound whole chicken
1 cinnamon stick
1 small onion, peeled
1 stalk of celery cut in half
3 bay leaves
2 whole black peppers
1 whole cardamom
1 teaspoon salt or to taste

Start to Finish
1 hour

Procedure

1• Clean and rinse chicken inside and out, then pat dry with a paper towel. Place chicken in a large pot, cover with water (about 8 cups), and bring to a boil over high heat.

2• Skim foam from the surface of the water and discard. Add remaining ingredients, stir, and reduce heat to medium-high. Cook 40 more minutes, turning the chicken once.

3• Turn off heat and transfer chicken onto a platter. Drain the broth through a fine sieve and set aside to cool.

4• Remove the fat from the top of the broth and discard. Debone the chicken. Broth and chicken are now ready to use in any recipe.

** TIP Chicken broth and chicken meat can be refrigerated up to 5 days or can be frozen up to a month.*

Nutrition Information per Serving

Calories 172, Fat 7g, Saturated fat 2g, Cholesterol 79mg, Carbohydrate 1g, Fiber 0g, Protein 26g

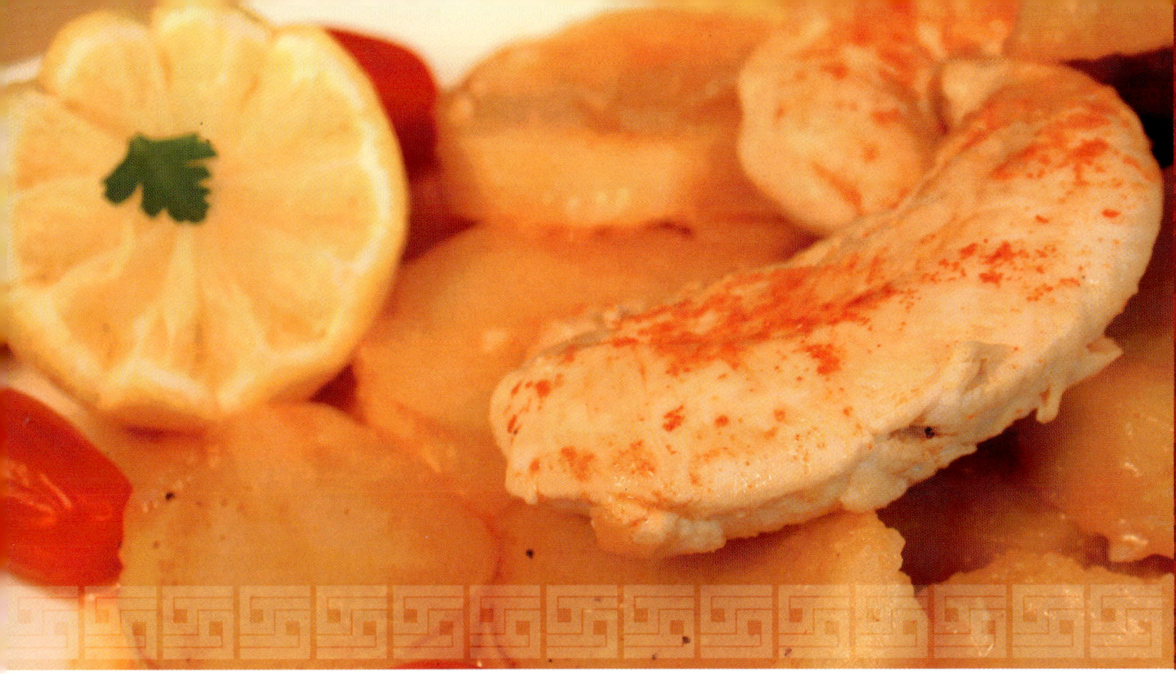

Chicken with Lemon & Garlic:

Dajaj b'Hamod w'Toom

دجاج بحامض وثوم

Ingredients

1½ pounds boneless, skinless chicken pieces
2 tablespoons vegetable oil
2 medium potatoes, peeled and cut into ¼-inch slices
½ teaspoon salt or to taste
½ teaspoon paprika

¾ cup fresh lemon juice
2 teaspoons minced garlic
¼ teaspoon salt
¼ cup water

Paper towels
Large skillet

Start to Finish
30 minutes
Serves 4

Procedure

1• Rinse and drain chicken pieces, and pat dry with a paper towel.

2• Pour oil into the skillet and place it over medium-high heat. Add chicken pieces and cook for several minutes or until golden brown.

3• Turn the chicken pieces and then add the sliced potatoes. Sprinkle with ½ teaspoon salt and paprika, cover, and cook for 5 minutes or until golden brown.

4• In a small bowl, combine lemon juice, garlic, salt and water; pour mixture all over the chicken and potatoes. Fold gently to bring potato pieces to the bottom of the skillet, cover and cook over medium heat for 5 more minutes.

Serve it hot or warm with pita bread and Salad.

** TIP Fresh chicken can be marinated for a couple of days in a covered container in the refrigerator.*

Nutrition Information per Serving

Calories 399, Fat 18.5g, Saturated fat 4g, Cholesterol 123mg, Carbohydrate 15g, Fiber 1g, Protein 41g

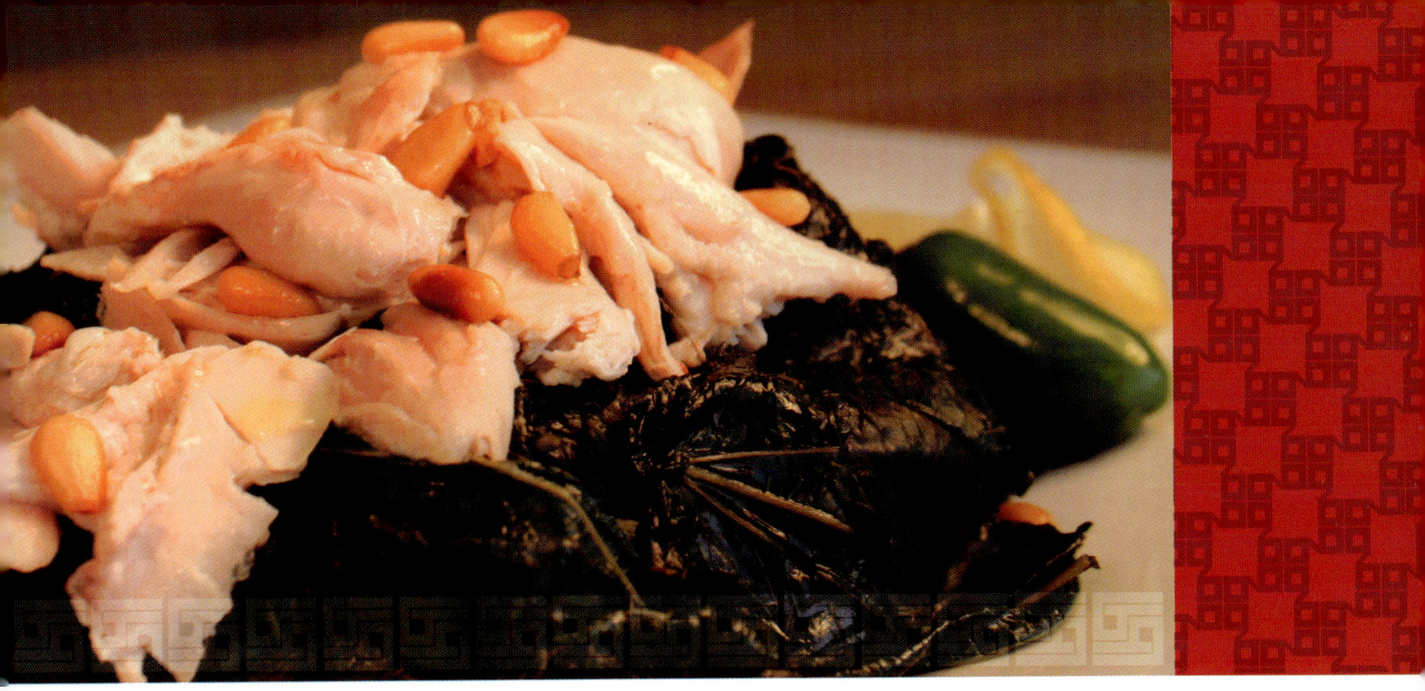

Molokhia is the green leaf of the jute plant. It can be bought fresh during the summer months, and dried or frozen year-round at any Middle Eastern market.

Chicken with Molokhia: Molokhia a Dajaj

دجاج وملوخيه

Ingredients

1 pound frozen molokhia, thawed
1 small onion, diced
2 tablespoons clarified butter
2 teaspoons crushed garlic
1 cup chopped cilantro, packed
¼ cup fresh lemon juice
¼ teaspoon ground seven spices

CHICKEN:
1 pound boneless, skinless chicken
1 cinnamon stick
2 bay leaves
1 teaspoon salt
¼ teaspoon ground white pepper
1 small onion, peeled

Start to Finish
30 minutes
Serves 6

Procedure

1• Place chicken in a medium-sized pot with water to cover and a bit more. Boil on high heat for 3 minutes.

2• Skim surface foam with a spoon and discard. Add cinnamon stick, bay leaves, salt, pepper and onion; stir, and reduce heat to medium-high.

3• Cook covered for 15 minutes, then turn off the heat. Remove chicken from pot, debone, and cut into small pieces. Strain broth with a fine sieve.

4• In the meantime, place butter in a large pot over high heat, add onion, and sauté for 5 minutes or until golden.

5• Stir in cilantro and garlic, and cook for 1 minute. Add molokhia, lemon juice and 3 cups strained chicken broth, and cook for 5 more minutes.

6• Add half of the chicken pieces to the pot and reduce heat to medium-low. Sprinkle with seven spices, stir, and cook covered for 5 more minutes.

7• Transfer to a platter, top with the remaining chicken pieces and serve.

Serve it hot with rice and lemon wedges, fresh onion, pickled hot peppers, cucumber pickles and fresh pita bread.

** TIP Cooked rice can be made on another burner while the molokhia is cooking.*

Nutrition Information per Serving

Calories 158, Fat 8g, Saturated fat 3.5g, Cholesterol 59mg, Carbohydrate 4g, Fiber 1g, Protein 17g

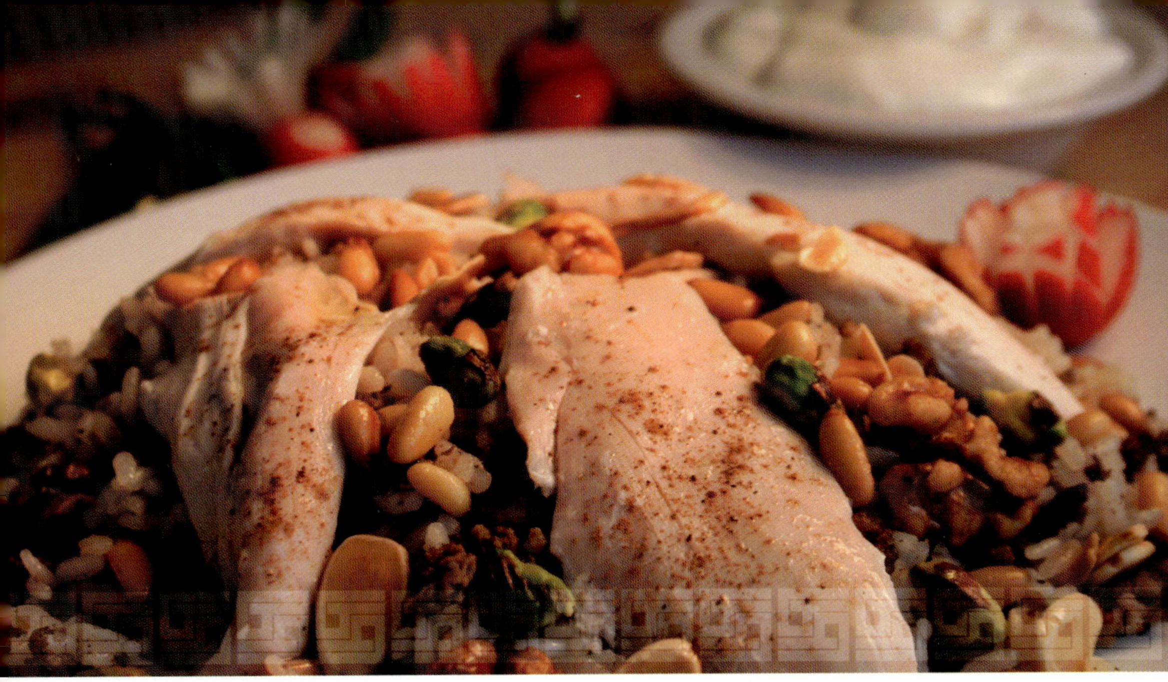

Chicken with Rice, Meat & Nuts:

Mansaf Dajaj

منسف دجاج

Ingredients

1 recipe cooked chicken, de-boned
(see Chicken Broth)

RICE:
3 cups medium grain rice, soaked and drained
3 cups warm water

NUTS:
¼ cup vegetable oil
¼ cup pine nuts
½ cup slivered almonds
¼ cup pistachio nuts
½ cup walnuts

MEAT:
1 small onion, finely chopped
1 pound ground lamb
1 teaspoon salt
½ teaspoon ground seven spices
¼ teaspoon ground cinnamon
¼ teaspoon ground black pepper

Slotted spoon
Paper towels

Start to Finish
30 minutes
plus De-bone chicken
Serves 8

Preparation

- De-bone chicken and set aside.

Procedure

1• Wash rice and soak it in water for 15 minutes, then drain.

2• Pour oil into a large pot over medium-high heat, stir in pine nuts, and sauté until they turn golden brown. (Be careful, they burn easily)

3• With a slotted spoon, remove pine nuts and spread them on a plate lined with paper towels to drain. Reserve oil in the pot.

4• Sauté almonds, pistachios and walnuts following the above steps. Again, reserve remaining oil in the pot.

5• Stir chopped onion into the remaining oil and sauté over high heat until golden brown.

6• Add ground meat and stir with a fork to separate while it cooks. Continue until the meat turns brown and moisture evaporates. Sprinkle salt, seven spices, cinnamon and black pepper over the meat. Stir in drained rice and cook until moisture evaporates, about 3 minutes.

7• Pour 3 cups water over rice and meat, stir, and bring to boil. When most of the water is absorbed, adjust salt to your taste and reduce heat to low; stir well, and cook covered for 12 minutes. Turn off heat and let it sit for 5 minutes.

8• Transfer cooked rice and meat to a large platter. Arrange chicken pieces on the top, and garnish with the toasted nuts.

Serve hot or warm with Yogurt Cucumber Salad or a salad of your choice.

** TIP De-boned chicken and meat can be done a couple of days in advance if kept refrigerated separately in a closed container.*

Nutrition Information per Serving

Calories 805, Fat 36g, Saturated fat 8g, Cholesterol 139mg, Carbohydrate 66g, Fiber 3g, Protein 52g

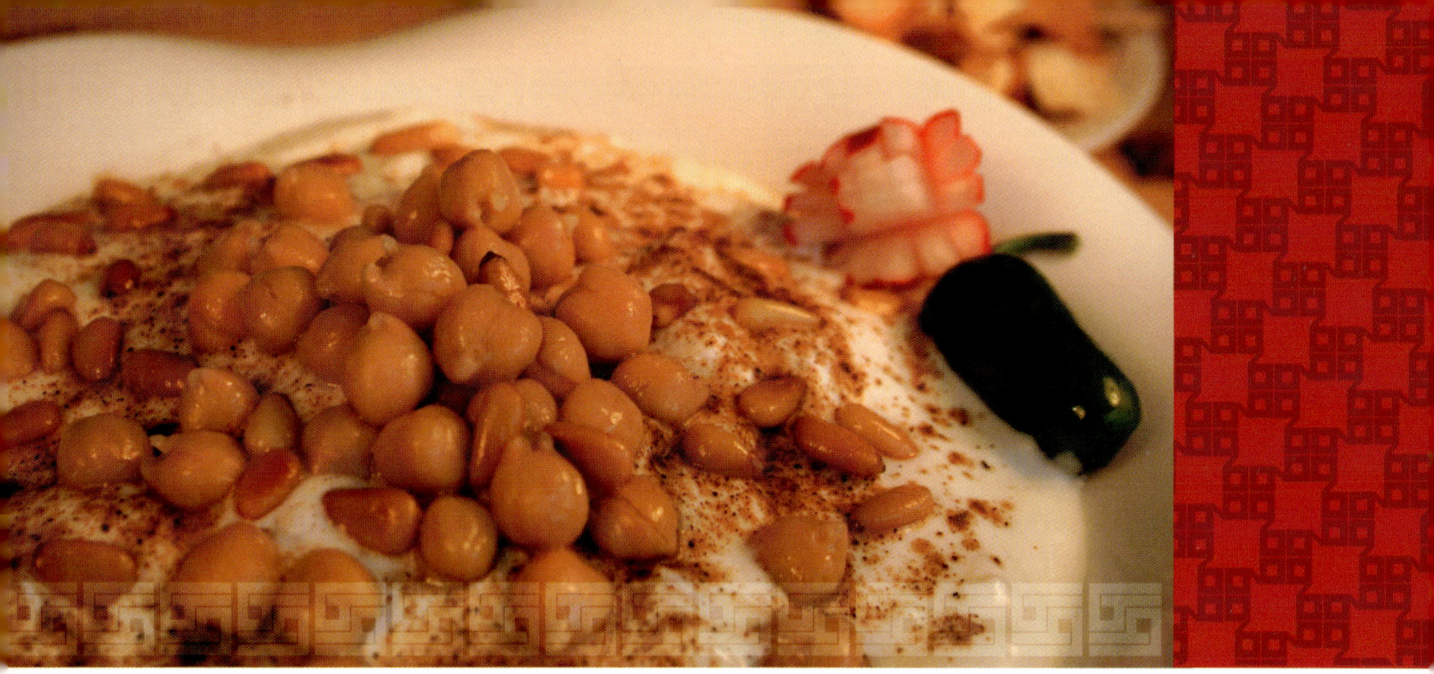

Topping the garlic-infused yogurt with pine nuts gives a special taste to this meal, and it is loaded with calcium.

Chick-peas with Bread & Yogurt:
Fattet Hummus

فتة حمص

Ingredients

2 cans chick-peas or
4 cups cooked chick-peas
2 cups water
½ teaspoon salt
¼ teaspoon allspice

11 x 7 x 1.5- inch pan
3 loaves pita bread cut into little pieces
2 tablespoons butter
¼ cup pine nuts

Yogurt Mixture:
4 cups plain yogurt
1 teaspoon crushed garlic
½ teaspoon salt or to taste

Start to Finish
20 minutes
Serves 8

Procedure

1• Wash canned chick-peas, drain and place in a medium pot with two cups water over high heat. Boil for 5 minutes, then turn to low, add salt, and cook covered for another 7 minutes or until the chick-peas are soft. Turn off heat and let covered pot sit, do not drain.

2• In the meantime, mix yogurt with garlic and salt and set aside.

3• Break pita bread into ¾-inch pieces and place them in the pan, then fold chick-peas and sauce into the bread, and level the surface with a spoon.

4• Spread yogurt evenly over chick-peas and bread. Sprinkle allspice on top.

5• Melt butter in a small pan over medium heat, stir in pine nuts and sauté until light golden brown, about one minute. (Be careful, they burn easily). Remove nuts from heat, pour over the yogurt topping and serve.

Serve it hot with scallions for breakfast, lunch, or dinner or as an appetizer.

***TIP** *Yogurt sauce can be prepared several days in advance.*

Nutrition Information per Serving

Calories 321, Fat 10g, Saturated fat 4g, Cholesterol 15mg, Carbohydrate 31g, Fiber 8g, Protein 17g

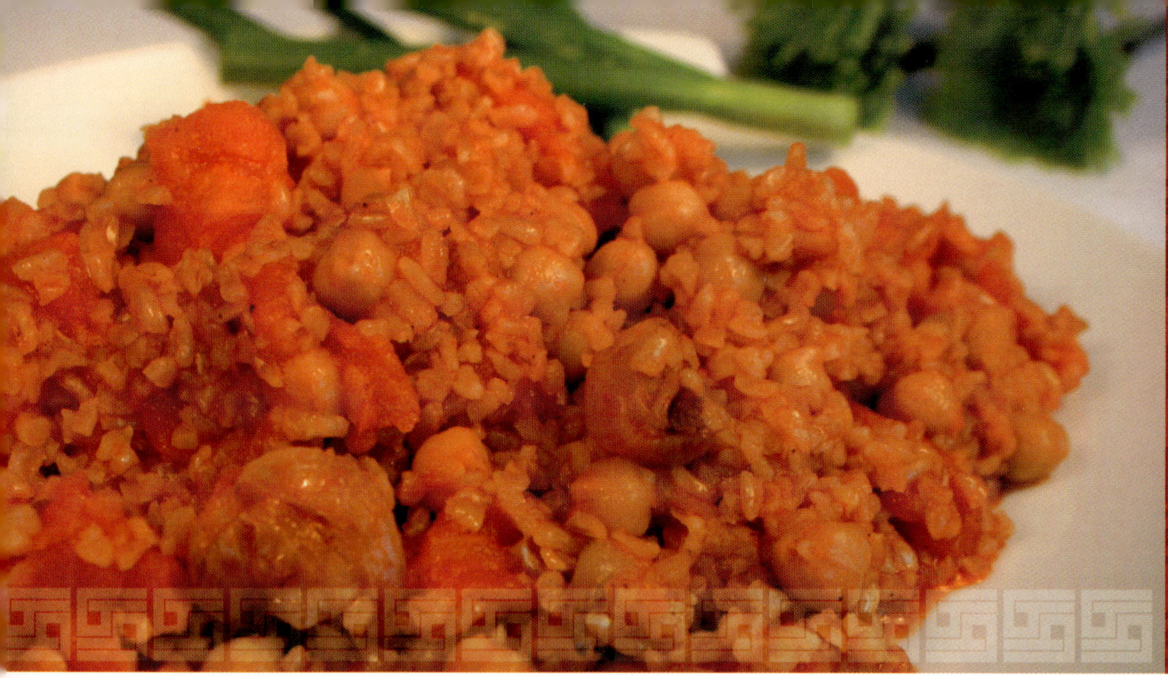

Cracked wheat or Burghul is important in the Lebanese diet; it is a delicious side dish as well as an easy main dish.

Cracked Wheat with Chick-peas:

Burghul bi' Dfeen

برغل بدفين

Ingredients

¼ cup olive oil
8 baby onions, peeled and cut in half
4 cups tomatoes, peeled and diced
1 cup chick-peas
1 cup cracked wheat # 4, washed and drained
1 teaspoon salt
⅛ teaspoon ground black pepper
⅛ teaspoon crushed hot pepper
2 cups water

Start to Finish
30 minutes
Serves 4

Procedure

1• Heat oil in a medium-sized pot on medium-high for 1 minute. Stir in onion and sauté until golden brown, about 3 minutes. Stir in tomatoes and sauté several more minutes. Fold in chick-peas.

2• Add drained cracked wheat, salt and black pepper to the pot, pour in water and bring to a boil.

3• Stir and cook until the water no longer looks soupy, but there is still a generous amount of liquid left. Cover pot, reduce heat to low and simmer for 10 minutes.

4• Turn off heat and let it sit for a few minutes before serving.

Serve it hot or warm with a salad of your choice.

** TIP This dish tastes best when it is freshly made. Meat and broth can be substituted for the tomato and water.*

Nutrition Information per Serving

Calories 451, Fat 14g, Saturated fat 2g, Cholesterol 0mg, Carbohydrate 69g, Fiber 18g, Protein 18g

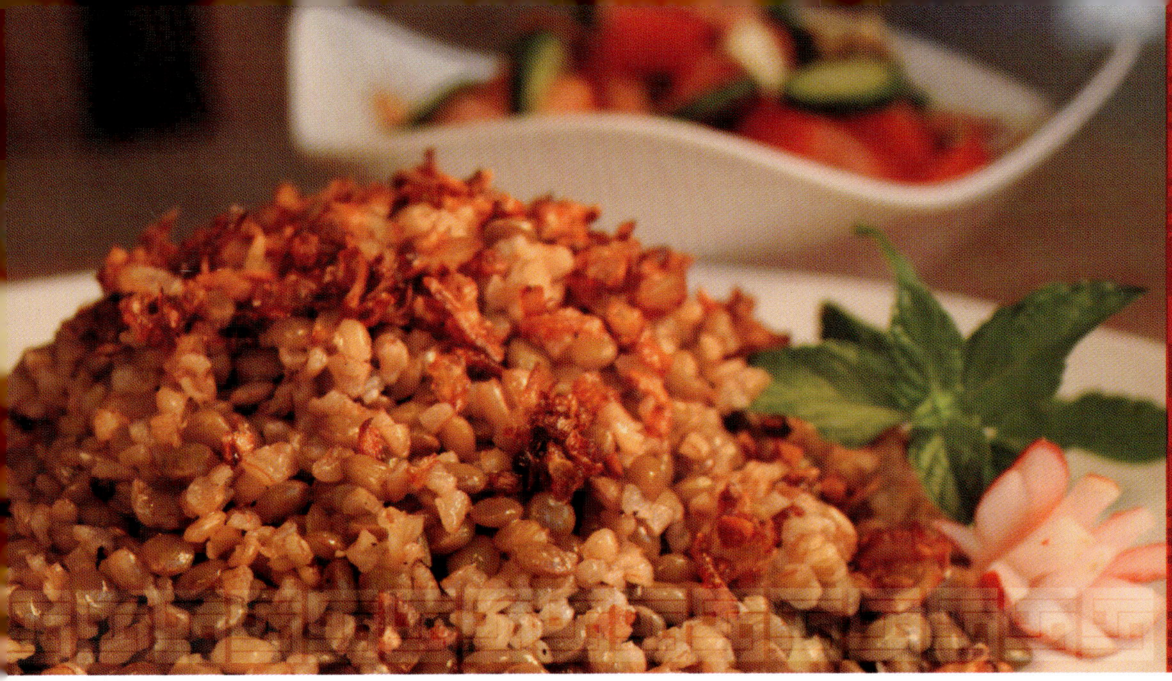

Cracked wheat with lentils is a general favorite in Lebanon. They call it aklet l'fou'kara or meal of the poor, because everyone can afford to make it.

Cracked Wheat with Lentils: M'jadrah

مجدره

Ingredients

1 cup lentils, sorted
⅓ cup olive oil
1 medium onion, finely chopped
1 cup cracked wheat (burghul #4), washed and drained
2¼ cups warm water
1 teaspoon salt or to taste
¼ teaspoon ground black pepper

Slotted spoon
Paper towels

Start to Finish
30 minutes
Serves 4

Procedure

1• Put lentils in a fine colander, wash and drain. Transfer to a medium pot, add water to cover and cook over high heat for 7 minutes.

2• Meanwhile, put oil in a saucepan over medium-high heat, stir in onion and sauté until medium brown. Turn off heat and remove onion with a slotted spoon to a platter lined with paper towels. Reserve hot oil in saucepan.

3• Add drained burghul to the lentils in the pot. Pour in 2¼ cups warm water and cook over medium-high heat until the liquid no longer looks soupy, but there is still a generous amount of liquid.

4• Sprinkle salt and pepper, stir, and reduce heat to low. Cover the pot and simmer for 15 more minutes.

5• Remove lid and pour reserved oil over the lentil mixture. Turn off heat and let it sit for a few minutes, then serve on a large platter and top with sautéed onions.

Serve it hot, warm or at room temperature with Toasted Bread Salad.

**TIP This tasty dish is loaded with iron and it refrigerates well up to a week. It is a great picnic dish!*

Nutrition Information per Serving

Calories 429, Fat 17g, Saturated fat 2g, Cholesterol 0mg, Carbohydrate 52g, Fiber 19g, Protein 20g

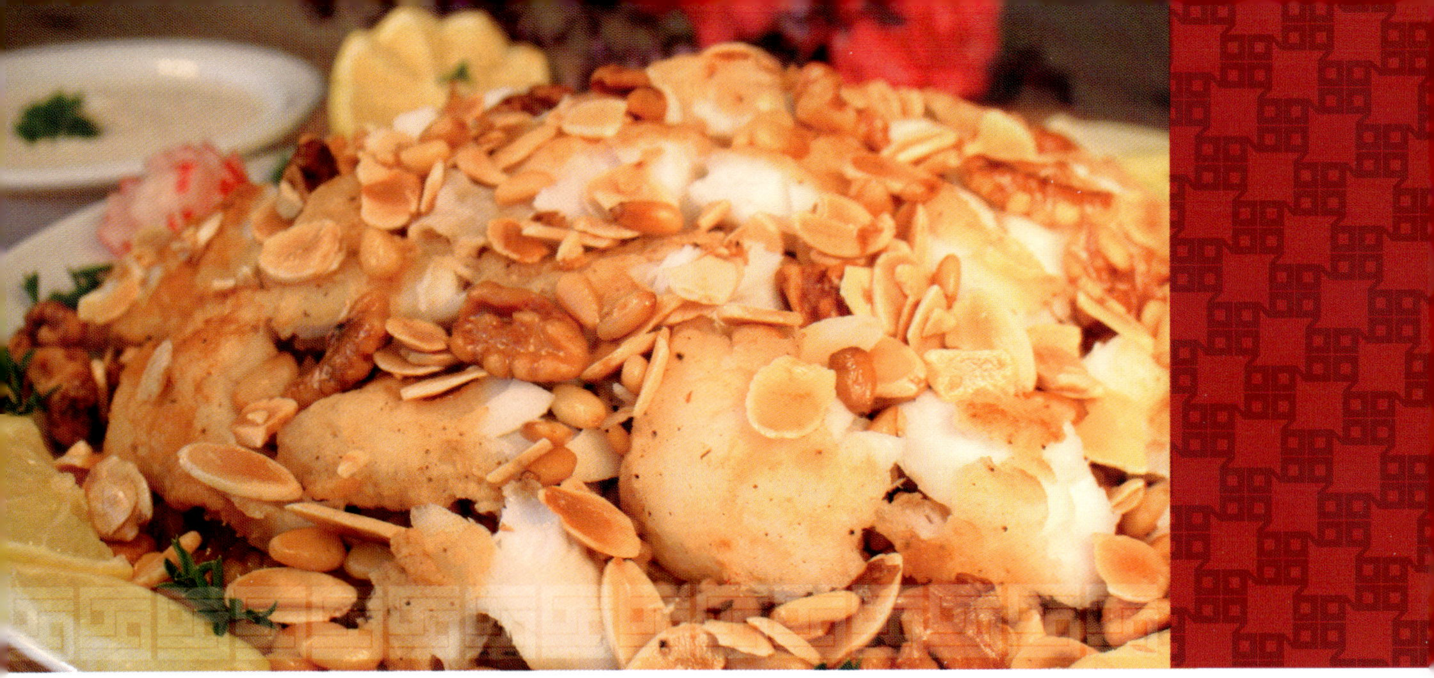

Fish are a big treat in Lebanon. Specialty fish restaurants can be found all along the coastal highway. One saltwater fish favored by the Lebanese is the red mullet (sultan ibrahim). Two of the most delectable dishes are samkeh harrah, a specialty of Tripoli, which is a large, whole baked fish served with tahini sauce, and sayadieh, which consists of brown seasoned rice with toasted nuts, topped by pieces of fried fish. Freshwater fish such as trout can be found in the river along the mountains. Fish are usually fried (my favorite) with ma'kalee, fried vegetables such as eggplant. They also can be baked or grilled and served with plain tahini sauce, tahini sauce and pine nuts or with cilantro and lemon garlic sauce.

Fish with Rice & Nuts: Sayadieh

صياديه

Ingredients

FISH:
2 pounds orange roughy fillets
2 cups vegetable oil
⅓ cup all-purpose flour
⅛ teaspoon cayenne
½ teaspoon salt or to taste
½ teaspoon seven spices
¼ teaspoon each cinnamon and paprika

RICE:
2 cups short grain rice, soaked and drained
¼ teaspoon ground cinnamon
¼ teaspoon ground black pepper
1 teaspoon salt or to taste

Large skillet and medium-sized pot
Fine sifter
Paper towels

ONION:
1 large onion, chopped
½ teaspoon salt
2 ¼ cups water

NUTS:
¼ cup pine nuts
½ cup slivered almonds
¼ cup pistachio nuts
½ cup walnuts

Start to Finish
30 minutes
Serves 6

Nutrition Information per Serving

Calories 534, Fat 27g, Saturated fat 2.5g, Cholesterol 29mg, Carbohydrate 44g, Fiber 3g, Protein 30g

Procedure

1• Put rice in a medium-sized bowl and rinse it 3 times or until the water runs clear. Soak rice in warm water for 10 minutes, then drain.

2• Put 2 cups vegetable oil in a large skillet over medium-high heat for 3 minutes. In the meantime, rinse fish and pat it dry with a paper towel. Combine flour, cayenne, salt, seven spices, cinnamon and paprika. Dip fish fillets in flour mixture one at a time to cover. Place floured fish in the hot oil and cook until they turn light golden brown on both sides. With a slotted spoon, transfer fish to a platter lined with paper towels to drain, and reserve hot oil.

3• Place medium-sized pot over medium-high heat, add ¼ cup of the hot fish oil, stir in onion and sauté until it is dark brown, but not burned.

4• With a slotted spoon, transfer 2 tablespoons of the cooked onion onto a plate lined with paper towels and set aside.

5• Add 2¼ cups water and ½ teaspoon salt to the remaining onion in the pot, boil it over high heat for 2 minutes, then turn off heat.

6• Use sifter to drain cooked onion over a bowl. Smash the onion in the sifter, drain well over the bowl and discard the remaining onion in the sifter. Pour the water in the bowl back into the pot and place over high heat. Add drained rice, cinnamon, pepper, 1 teaspoon salt and 2 tablespoons of the fish oil. Stir, and bring to a boil for several minutes.

7• Reduce heat to medium and stir briefly. When most of the liquid is absorbed, reduce heat to low, stir, and cook covered for 10 minutes, then turn off heat and let it sit for 5 minutes.

8• Meanwhile, toast each type of nut separately in the fish oil over medium-high heat. (Be careful, they burn quickly). With a slotted spoon, transfer nuts to a plate lined with paper towels and discard the fish oil.

9• Spoon cooked rice onto a large platter and fluff it with a fork. Break the fish into pieces and arrange on top of the rice, then garnish the surface with the toasted nuts.

Serve it hot or warm with Tahini Sauce with Pine Nuts, hummus and salad.

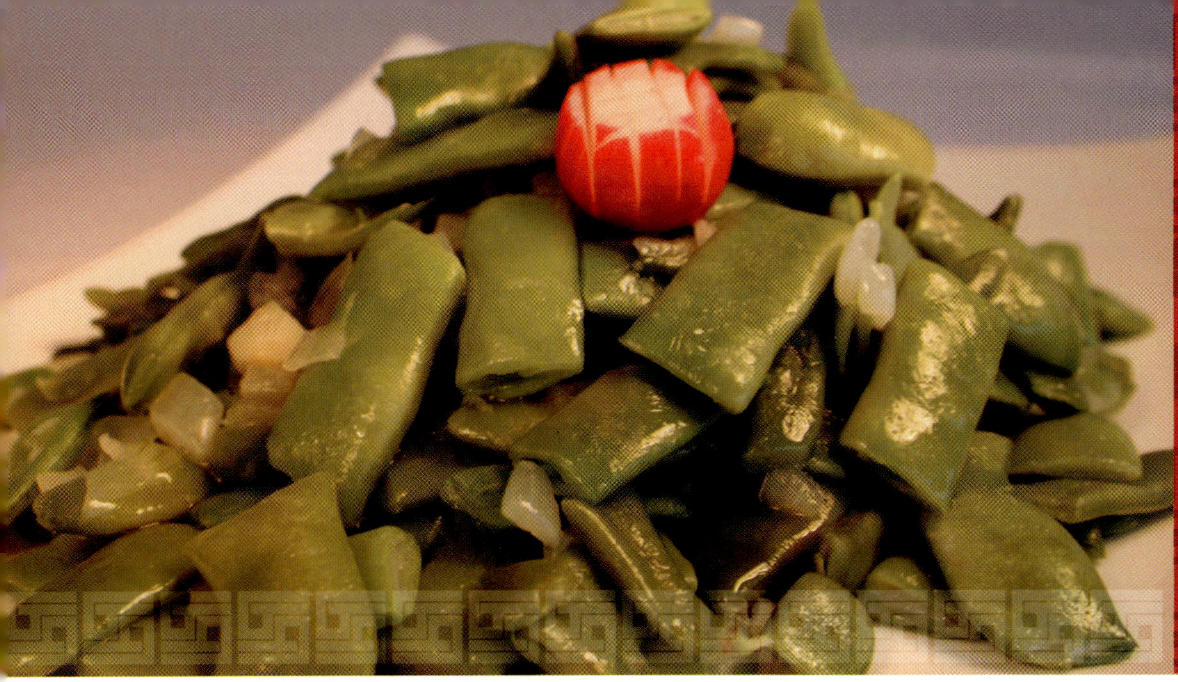

Green beans can be served as an appetizer or as a side dish. Eat them by hand with torn pieces of bread, or with a fork.

Green Beans: Loubieh b'Zeit

لوبيه بزيت

Ingredients

1 pound frozen Italian green beans, thawed
3 tablespoons olive oil
1 small onion, chopped
½ teaspoon sugar
2 tablespoons water
1 teaspoon salt
⅛ teaspoon ground black pepper

Start to Finish
30 minutes
Serves 2-4

Procedure

1• Place oil in a medium-sized skillet over medium-high heat, stir in onion and sauté for 5 minutes. Add sugar and stir briefly.

2• Combine beans with the onion, add 2 tablespoons water, and cook covered for 10 minutes, stirring frequently.

3• Uncover skillet, sprinkle salt and pepper, stir, then replace the lid. Reduce heat to medium-low and cook for 10 minutes or until beans are tender.

4• Turn off heat and transfer to a serving platter.

Serve it warm, at room temperature or cold with Lebanese Spaghetti and salad.

**TIP Green beans can be cooked a few days in advance. Adding diced tomato and garlic to the green beans makes them even tastier. Also meat can be added.*

Nutrition Information per Serving

Calories 241, Fat 17g, Saturated fat 8g, Cholesterol 70mg, Carbohydrate 6g, Fiber 2g, Protein 15g

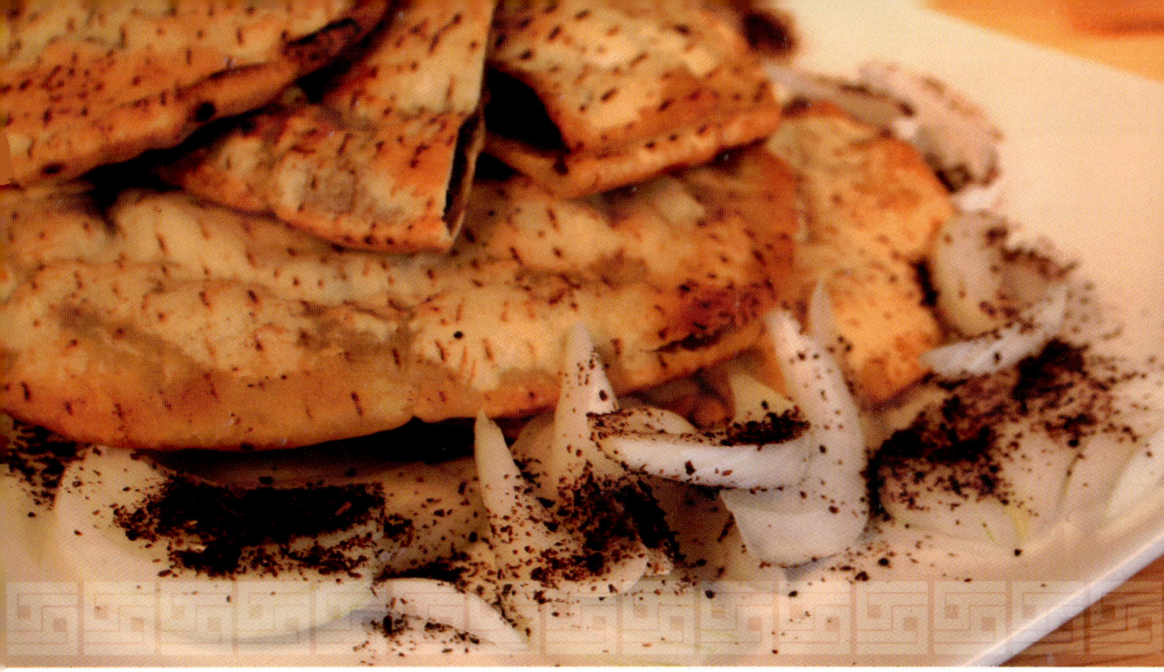

Arayes Kafta is one of the finest and easiest of Lebanese appetizers. It can also be enjoyed as the main dish of a delicious meal.

Kafta in Pita Bread: Arayes Kafta

عرايس كفته

Ingredients

1 recipe kafta (see kafta kebabs)
8 loaves small pita bread
3 tablespoons vegetable oil

Three 11- x 13-inch pans
1 small onion, sliced into thin wedges
1 tablespoon sumac

Start to Finish
30 minutes
Serves 4

Procedure

1• Preheat oven to 400 degrees F.

2• Open each loaf of bread ¾ of the way, so that the two layers are still attached from one side.

3• Place ⅓ cup kafta on each bottom layer, spread it with a spoon, and cover it with the top layer.

4• Brush the filled sandwiches on both sides with oil. Cut them in half so that the top and bottom layers are still attached, and arrange them in the pans.

5• Bake for 10 minutes, then rotate the pans and turn over all the sandwiches. Return them to the oven for 5 more minutes, or until golden brown.

6• Combine sliced onion and sumac and spread on a large platter. Arrange cooked Arayes Kafta over the onion and serve.

Serve it hot with Yogurt Cucumber Salad or hummus.

***TIP** *Bread may be brushed with butter instead of oil.*

Nutrition Information per Serving

Calories 407, Fat 17g, Saturated fat 5.5g, Cholesterol 75mg, Carbohydrate 34g, Fiber 2g, Protein 27g

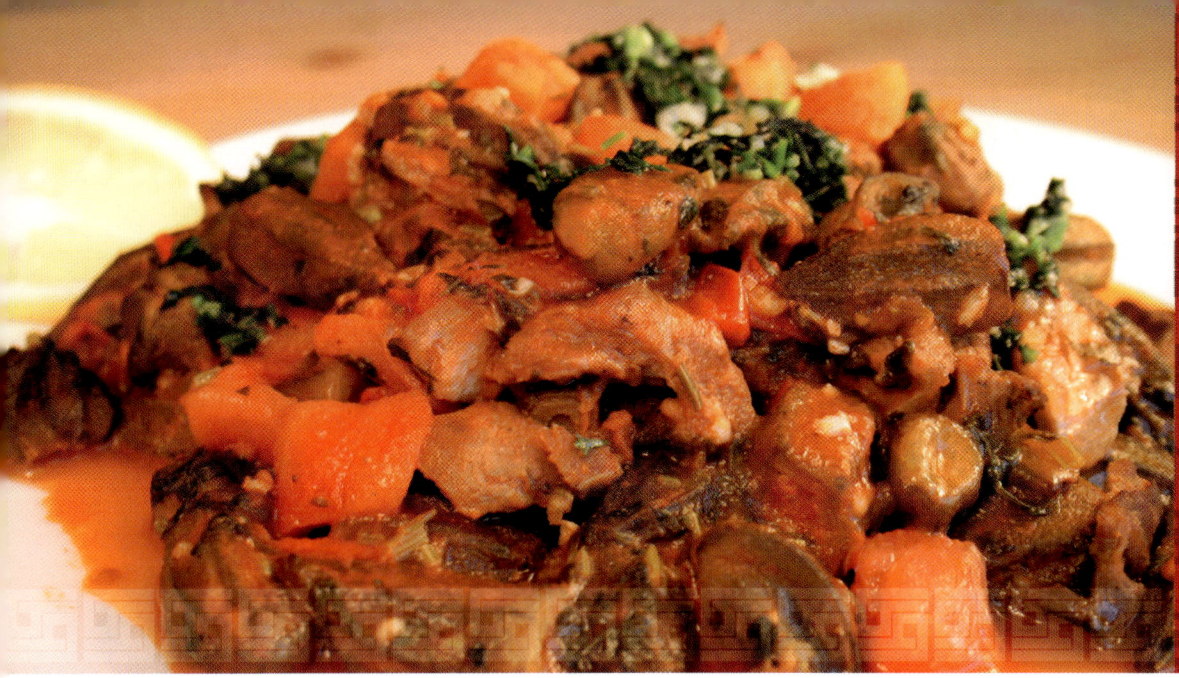

Stews (Al Yakhani البخاني) are the foundation for a number of nourishing daily meals. They begin with meat and vegetables, which can be cooked simply with onion and water, or accented with fresh tomatoes, tomato sauce, yogurt sauce, or a cilantro-garlic sauce. Lebanese stews are regularly served with plain rice, rice with lentils or vermicelli rice, a delicious variation.

Lamb Stew with Baby Okra:

Bamieh b'Lahmeh

بامیه بلحمه

Ingredients

1 pound frozen baby okra, thawed
1 tablespoon vegetable oil
1 tablespoon clarified butter
1 pound extra lean lamb, cut into small pieces
¼ teaspoon ground black pepper
¼ teaspoon ground seven spices
⅛ teaspoon cinnamon
2 cups peeled tomatoes cut into 1-inch cubes
1 cup tomato sauce
2 cups water
1 teaspoon salt
2 tablespoons vegetable oil
1 bunch fresh cilantro, washed and finely chopped
1 tablespoon minced garlic

Preheat oven to 450 degrees F.
Paper towels
Large baking pan for okra

Start to Finish
30 minutes
Serves 6

Procedure

1• Pat dry okra with paper towels, place in baking pan and coat with 1 tablespoon oil. Bake in oven for 10 minutes or until they are golden, stirring once.

2• Meanwhile, melt clarified butter in a large skillet over medium-high heat, stir in lamb pieces and sauté for 7 minutes. Sprinkle lamb with pepper, seven spices, and cinnamon, then add cubed tomatoes and sauté for 5 more minutes

3• Stir in tomato sauce and water and heat to boiling. Add cooked okra, stir, and cover. Reduce heat to medium and cook for 10 minutes.

4• Meanwhile, heat 2 tablespoons oil in a pan on medium-high heat, stir in chopped cilantro and crushed garlic, and sauté for 1 minute. Add this mixture to the stew, stir, and cook for another minute.

5• Remove from heat. Transfer to a deep platter and serve.

Serve it hot or warm with Rice with Vermicelli, fresh pita bread and scallions.

** TIP The okra can be baked a few days in advance.*

Nutrition Information per Serving

Calories 284, Fat 21g, Saturated fat 7g, Cholesterol 59mg, Carbohydrate 9g, Fiber 3g, Protein 16g

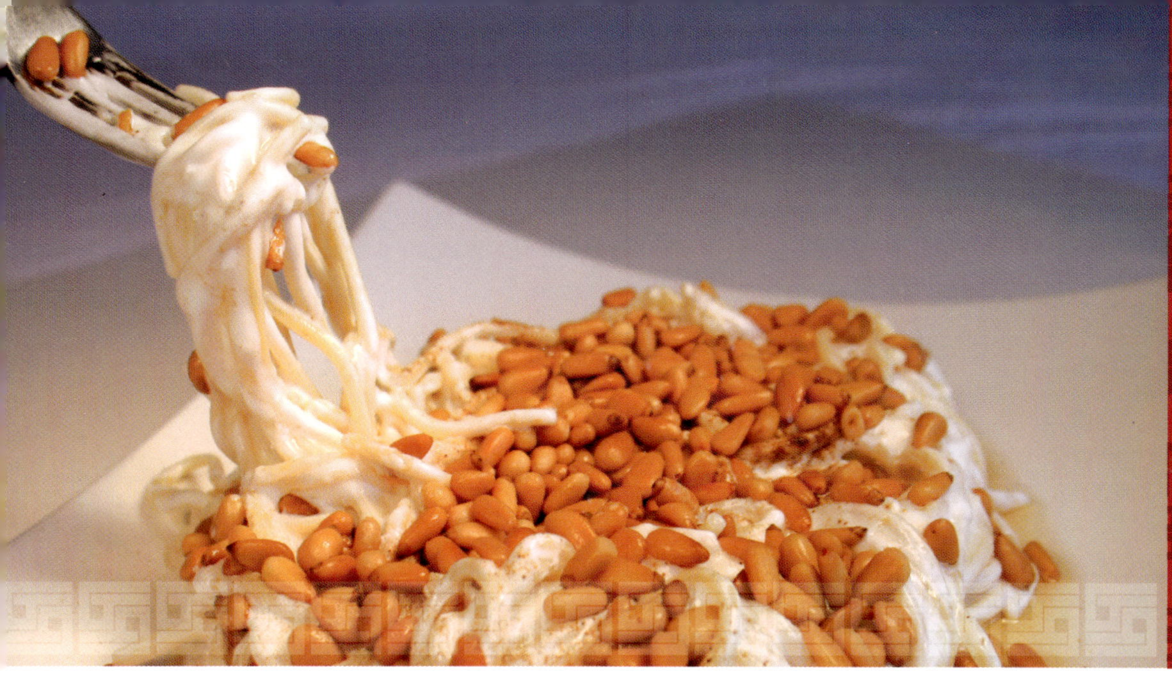

Hurry up-and Serve it up.
Safa Merheb dresses cooked spaghetti in garlic-infused yogurt, then tops it with spicy cooked meat and a sprinkling of pine nuts toasted in butter.
Arizona Daily Star F1-NE /Wednesday October 9, 2002

Lebanese Spaghetti: Macarona b'Laban

معكرونه باللبن

Ingredients

One (16-ounce) package of spaghetti
¼ teaspoon seven spices
2 tablespoons butter
1 tablespoon vegetable oil
⅓ cup pine nuts

Yogurt Mixture:

4 cups plain yogurt
1 teaspoon crushed garlic
½ teaspoon salt or to taste

Start to Finish
20 minutes
Serves 6

Procedure

1• Break spaghetti into thirds and cook according to package directions.

2• Meanwhile, add the crushed garlic and salt to the yogurt, stir well, and set aside.

3• When the spaghetti is done, drain well and place in a large serving dish. Add yogurt mixture to the spaghetti, toss gently, and sprinkle seven spices over the top.

4• Place butter and 1 tablespoon oil in a pan over medium-high heat. When butter is melted, add pine nuts. Stir until pine nuts are light golden brown, being careful not to burn them.

5• Turn off the heat and pour nut mixture evenly over the top.

Serve it hot or warm with Green Beans and salad.

** TIP Adults and children love this dish! You can also top it with meat and pine nuts.*

Nutrition Information per Serving

Calories 425, Fat 13g, Saturated fat 5g, Cholesterol 20mg, Carbohydrate 58g, Fiber 3g, Protein 18g

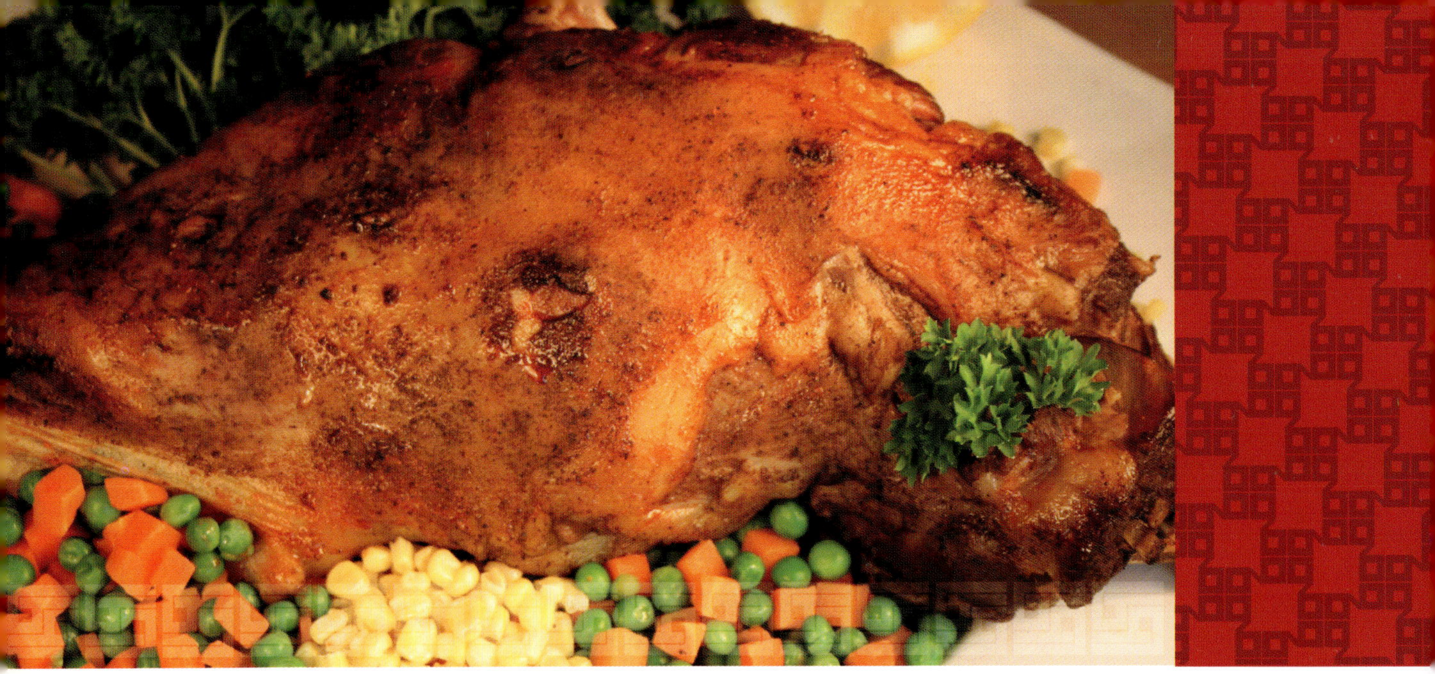

The aromatic smell and taste and the tender, juicy, texture of lamb is present whether you bake or barbecue it.

Baked Leg of Lamb: Fakhed Ghanam bil Furn

فخد غنم بالفرن

Ingredients

4 to 5-pound leg of lamb
1 tablespoon salt
1 teaspoon ground seven spices
1 teaspoon ground black pepper
1 teaspoon cinnamon
¼ teaspoon cardamom
7 cloves garlic, peeled
1 tablespoon vegetable oil
1 large onion, quartered
2 cups baby carrots

13¼ x 9½ x 2¼-inch pan
Aluminum foil

Preparation

- Pat the leg of lamb dry with a paper towel and place in the pan.
- Mix salt, seven spices, black pepper, cinnamon and cardamom. Sprinkle it over the leg of lamb and rub in gently with your hands.
- With a knife, make 7 slits in the leg of lamb, 4 on top and 3 at the bottom. Place a clove of garlic in each slit.
- Coat the meat with vegetable oil and set aside.

To Garnish

- parsley and lemon wedges

SAUCE:
Juice from the cooked leg of lamb
2 tablespoons flour
1 tablespoon cornstarch
1/8 teaspoon seven spices
1/8 teaspoon cardamom
2 cups warm water

Start to Finish
5 minutes
without baking
Serves 10

Nutrition Information
per Serving

Calories 387, Fat 26g, Saturated fat 11g, Cholesterol 115mg, Carbohydrate 6g, Fiber 1g, Protein 30g

Procedure

1• Place the leg of lamb in the oven at 450 degrees F. for one hour.

2• Remove pan from oven, turn over the leg of lamb, and return it to the oven to cook 15 more minutes.

3• Remove the leg of lamb from the oven, turn it over again, and place onion and carrots around it. Cover the pan with foil and return it to the oven to bake for 30 minutes.

4• Take pan out of the oven, remove foil, and baste the leg of lamb. Decrease oven temperature to 350 degrees F. Return pan to the oven to bake uncovered for half an hour, basting twice.

5• Remove pan from oven and let it sit for 10 minutes. Transfer leg of lamb and vegetables onto a large platter and garnish with parsley and lemon wedges. Reserve juice in the pan.

6• Place juice in a saucepan over medium-high heat. Combine flour, corn starch, spice and cardamom. Slowly add them to the juice while stirring with a wire whisk. Continue to stir for several minutes.

7• Slowly add water while whisking until the sauce is smooth. Adjust salt and thickness as desired. Serve sauce aside the leg of lamb.

Serve it hot with steamed vegetables and with rice and nuts.

** TIP Leg of Lamb can be prepared for baking a couple of days in advance if kept in the refrigerator.*

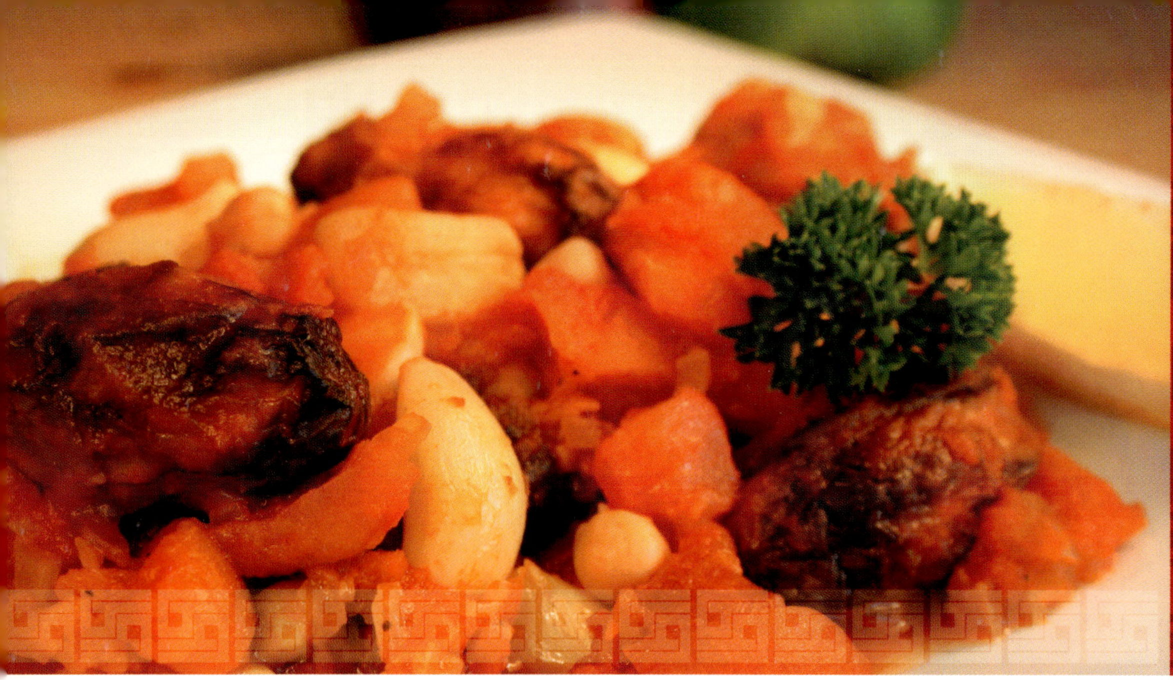

Moussaka: Moussaka'it Bazenjaan

مصقعة باذنجان

Ingredients

2 eggplants, peeled and cut into 8 thick wedges or 8 baby eggplants
½ teaspoon salt
2 tablespoons vegetable oil
1 medium onion, diced
½ cup peeled whole garlic
1 teaspoon salt
2 cups tomatoes, peeled and diced
2 tablespoons fresh lemon juice
1½ cups cooked chick-peas
¼ teaspoon ground black pepper
1 cup water

Deep fryer
2 cups vegetable oil
Paper towels
Large skillet

Start to Finish
30 minutes
Serves 4 - 6

Procedure

1• Place eggplant wedges on a paper towel and sprinkle with ½ teaspoon salt. Let them sit for 5 minutes, then pat dry with paper towels.

2• Pour oil in the deep fryer and heat on high for 3 minutes.

3• Gently place eggplant wedges in the hot oil to fry until they are golden brown on all sides, then remove them with a slotted spoon and drain on a paper towel.

4• Meanwhile, put 2 tablespoons vegetable oil in a large skillet over medium-high heat, stir in diced onion and sauté for several minutes. Add garlic and sauté for 3 more minutes. Sprinkle onion and garlic with salt, stir in tomato and lemon juice, and sauté another 5 minutes.

5• Add chickpeas, sprinkle with pepper, and pour in 1 cup water. Bring to a boil and gently add drained eggplant. Reduce heat to medium and cook for 5 minutes, turning eggplant wedges once.

6• Turn off heat and transfer to a deep platter to serve.

Serve it hot, warm or cold with fresh pita bread or by itself as an appetizer.

**TIP The eggplant can be fried a couple of days in advance.*
A 15-ounce can of garbanzo beans can be substituted for the cooked chickpeas.
Meat lovers can add Meat with Pine Nuts to it.

Nutrition Information per Serving

Calories 199, Fat 6g, Saturated fat 1g, Cholesterol 0mg, Carbohydrate 32g, Fiber 11g, Protein 7g

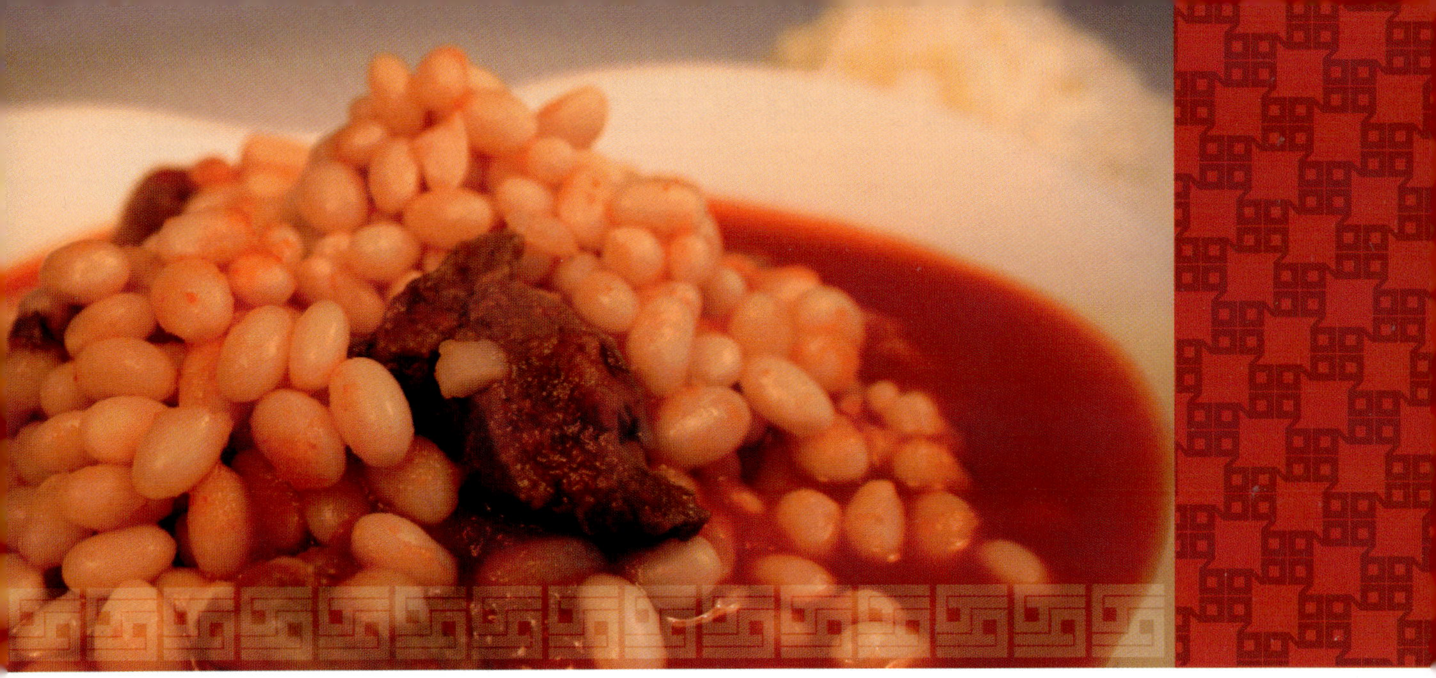

This is a favorite meal for everyone; the lamb gives it a delicious taste, but it can be made with another meat of your choice.

Navy Bean & Lamb Stew: Fasolia b'Lahmeh

فاصوليا بلحمه

Ingredients

1 pound dry navy beans
1 medium onion, finely chopped
¼ cup clarified butter
1 pound stewing lamb, cut into small pieces
2 cups tomato sauce
1 teaspoon salt or to taste
¼ teaspoon ground seven spices
⅛ teaspoon ground black pepper
⅛ teaspoon ground cinnamon

Pressure pot

Start to Finish
30 minutes
Serves 6

Preparation

• Sort and wash beans in a colander under cold running water, then place them in the pressure pot with 7 cups of water to soak overnight.

Procedure

1• The next day, bring the pressure pot to a boil over high heat and discard any foam from the top.

2• Meanwhile, melt clarified butter in a large pan over medium-high heat, stir in onion, and sauté for several minutes. Add meat and cook until it browns, about 5 minutes.

3• Pour meat mixture into the boiling beans and stir in tomato sauce, salt, seven spices, pepper and cinnamon. Pressurize pot according to directions in the manual.

4• When the pressure pot starts to whistle, reduce heat to medium and cook for 15 minutes. Turn off heat and follow directions in the manual to open the pressure pot. Adjust salt and serve beans in a deep bowl.

Serve it hot with fresh bread and Rice with Vermicelli.

** TIP The rice can be prepared while the beans are cooking. Chopped cilantro and crushed garlic can be added to the navy beans.*

Nutrition Information per Serving

Calories 389, Fat 17g, Saturated fat 8g, Cholesterol 67mg, Carbohydrate 34g, Fiber 9g, Protein 25g

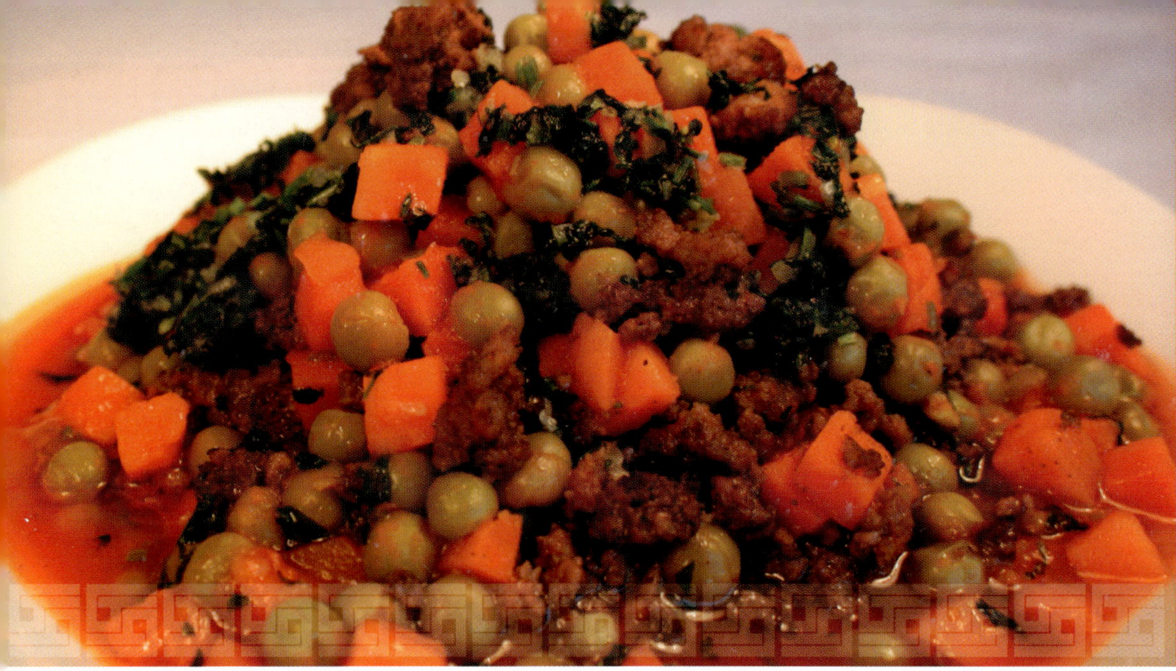

Pea Stew with Cilantro: Yakhnit Bazilla

يخنة بازيلا

Ingredients

½ pound ground meat
2 tablespoons clarified butter
¼ teaspoon seven spices
⅛ teaspoon cinnamon
⅛ teaspoon black pepper
½ teaspoon salt
½ bunch cilantro, washed and finely chopped
1 clove crushed garlic
1 pound frozen peas and carrots, thawed
1 cup tomato sauce
2 cups water
½ teaspoon salt or to taste
⅛ teaspoon pepper

Medium pot

Start to Finish
30 minutes
Serves 4

Procedure

1• Melt clarified butter in the pot over high heat, add meat, and stir with a fork to separate. Cook for 5 minutes or until moisture evaporates. Sprinkle meat with seven spices, cinnamon, pepper, and salt.

2• Stir in chopped cilantro and crushed garlic and cook for one minute. Add peas and carrots, and continue to sauté several more minutes.

3• Pour in tomato sauce and water, stir, and boil for 5 minutes.

4• Reduce heat to medium, add salt and pepper, and cook covered for 10 more minutes. Remove from heat and serve.

Serve it hot with Rice with Vermicelli, fresh pita bread and salad.

** TIP Rice can be prepared on another burner while the stew is cooking.*

Nutrition Information per Serving

Calories 234, Fat 13g, Saturated fat 6g, Cholesterol 53mg, Carbohydrate 17g, Fiber 5g, Protein 15g

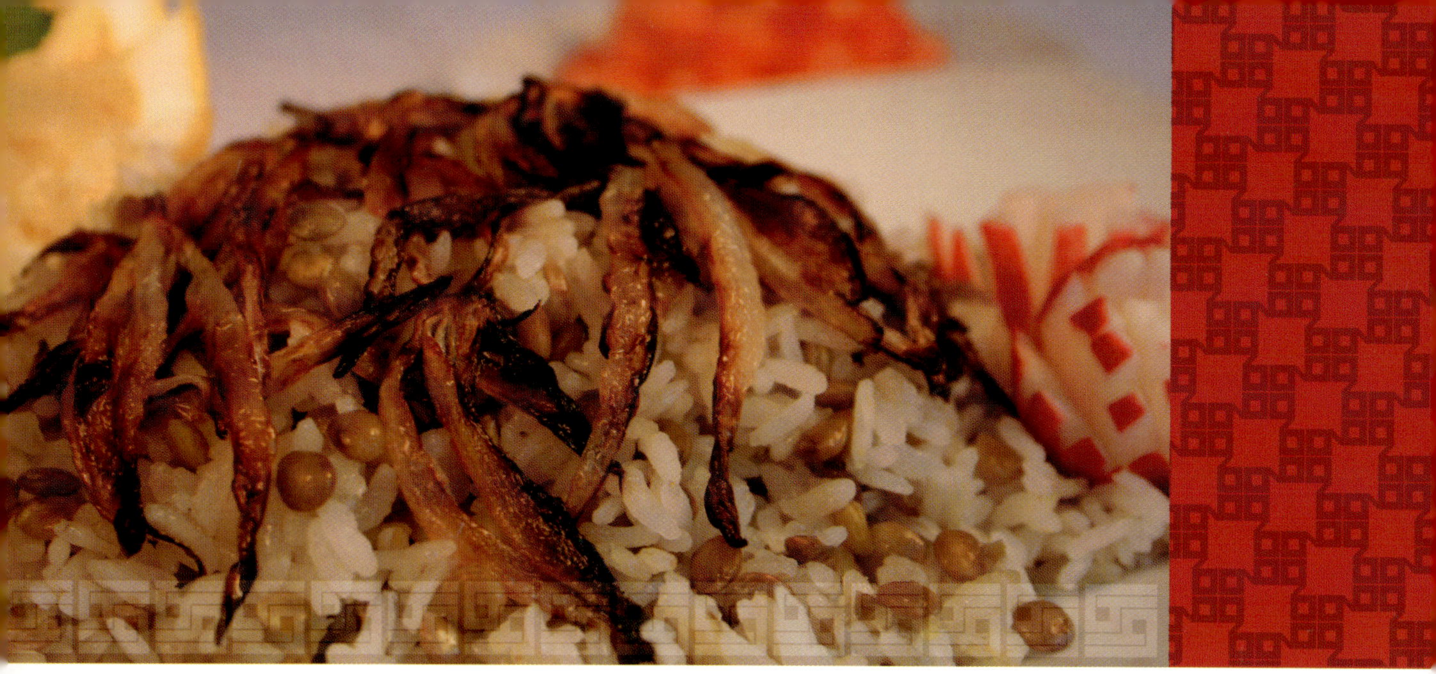

Rice with Lentils: M'dardarit Riz w'Adas

مدردرة رز وعدس

Ingredients

2 cups short grain rice
1 cup lentils, sorted
1 teaspoon salt or to taste
¼ teaspoon ground black pepper

⅓ cup olive oil or vegetable oil
1 large onion, sliced into thin wedges

Start to Finish
30 minutes
Serves 6

Preparation

• Put rice in a fine colander and fit it over a large bowl. Rinse rice until the water running into the bowl is clear, then remove the colander to drain the rice. Discard the water. Place drained rice in the empty bowl with 3 cups hot water and soak for 10 minutes.

Procedure

1• Put lentils in a fine colander and rinse well. Place them in a medium pot with 2 cups water over high heat for 5 minutes.

2• Reduce heat to medium, stir, and cover. Cook for 5 more minutes, then add the soaked rice and water to the lentils.

3• Raise heat to high and cook for 5 minutes or until most of the liquid is absorbed.

4• Add salt and pepper, and stir well. Reduce heat to low, cover, and cook for 15 minutes.

5• Meanwhile, put oil in a pan over medium-high heat, add onion, and sauté until medium brown.

6• Remove cooked onion with a slotted spoon to a plate layered with paper towels. Reserve hot oil.

7• Uncover the pot, pour reserved hot oil over cooked rice and lentils, and gently fold with a spoon. Replace cover and let it sit for a few minutes before transferring to a serving platter. Fluff the top with a fork and garnish with onion before serving.

Serve it hot or warm with Yogurt Cucumber Salad.

** TIP This side dish refrigerates well in a covered container for a week.*

Nutrition Information per Serving

Calories 503, Fat 11g, Saturated fat 1g, Cholesterol 0mg, Carbohydrate 83g, Fiber 11g, Protein 17g

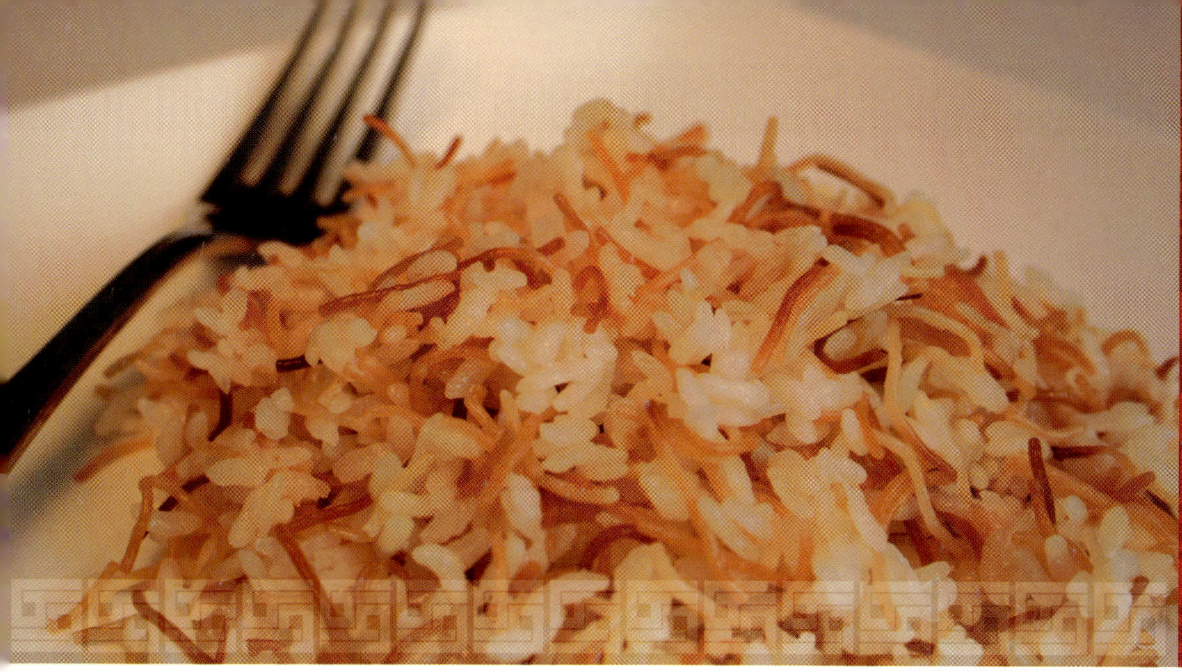

Rice with Vermicelli: Riz bi'Shayrieh

رز بشعيريه

Ingredients

2 cups short grain rice
4 cups water
3 tablespoons clarified butter
1 cup vermicelli
1 teaspoon salt or to taste

Start to Finish
20 minutes
plus soaking time
Serves 6

Preparation

• Put rice in a fine colander and fit it over a large bowl. Rinse rice until the water running into the bowl is clear, then remove the colander to drain the rice. Discard the water. Place drained rice in the empty bowl with 4 cups warm water and soak for 15 minutes.

Procedure

1• Melt butter in a medium pot over high heat. Add vermicelli, stir, and cook until golden brown. (Be careful, it burns easily).

2• Add soaked rice and the water, stir, and bring to boil for 5 minutes or until most of the liquid is absorbed.

3• Add salt and stir. Reduce heat to low, cover, and cook for 10 minutes.

4• Turn off heat and let it sit for a few minutes. When ready to serve, gently fold rice and vermicelli and transfer to a platter. Fluff the top with a fork.

Serve it hot or warm with stew, vegetables, or by itself with plain yogurt.

** TIP Vegetable oil can be substituted for the clarified butter.*

Nutrition Information per Serving

Calories 314, Fat 5g, Saturated fat 1g, Cholesterol 0mg, Carbohydrate 61g, Fiber 0g, Protein 5g

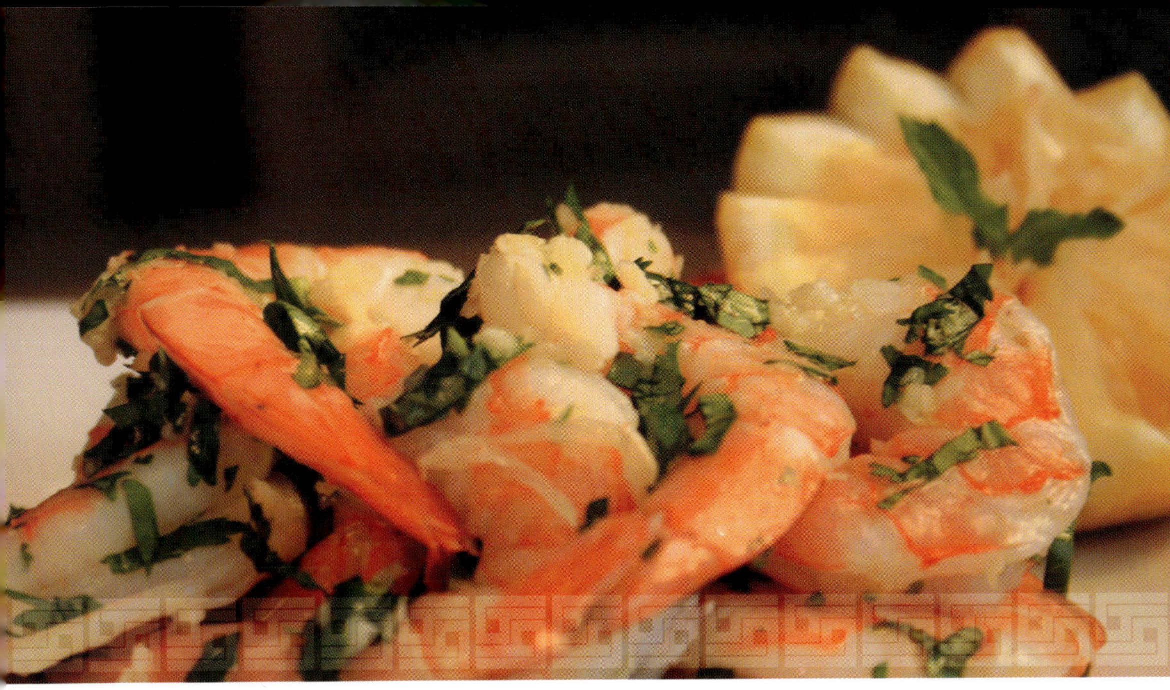

Shrimp with Cilantro & Garlic:

A'raydes b'Kizibra w'Toom

قريدس بكزبره وثوم

Ingredients

1 pound medium, raw shrimp, shelled and de-veined
1 bunch cilantro, washed and finely chopped
2 tablespoons crushed garlic
½ teaspoon salt or to taste
¼ teaspoon allspice
⅛ teaspoon cayenne
¼ teaspoon celery salt
¼ cup olive oil
1 small onion, chopped
1 cup water

Start to Finish
20 minutes
Serves 4

Procedure

1• On a large platter, combine shelled shrimp, chopped cilantro, crushed garlic, salt, allspice, cayenne and celery salt then set aside.

2• Place oil in a large skillet over medium heat, stir in chopped onion and sauté until golden. Stir in shrimp mixture and sauté until shrimp turns pink. Add water, bring to a boil and cook for 5 more minutes, then turn off heat and serve.

Serve it hot or warm as an appetizer or with rice as a main dish.

** TIP Shrimp can be marinated with cilantro and garlic overnight if refrigerated in a covered container.*

Nutrition Information per Serving

Calories 249, Fat 15g, Saturated fat 2g, Cholesterol 166mg, Carbohydrate 4g, Fiber 1g, Protein 23g

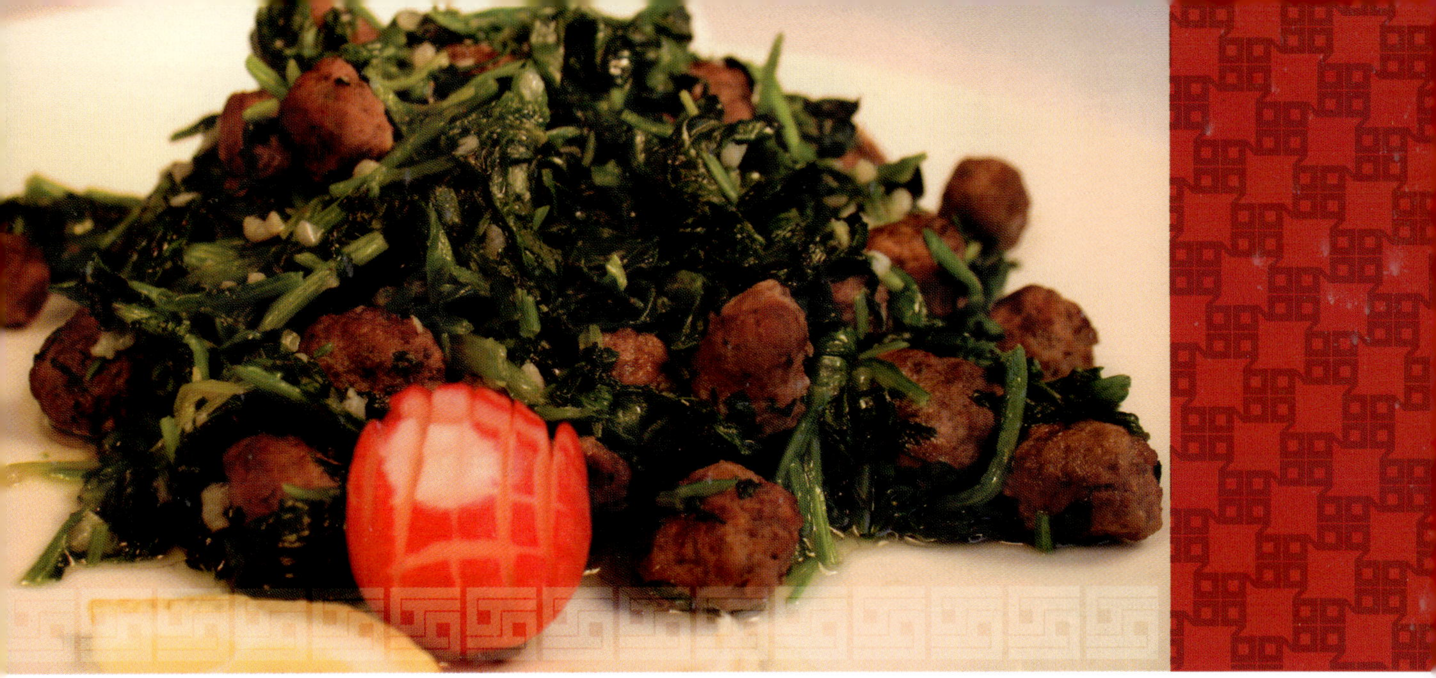

Spinach Stew: Yakhnit Sabaneikh

يخنة سبانخ

Ingredients

1 pound frozen baby spinach, thawed
1 pound ground meat
1 teaspoon salt
¼ teaspoon seven spices
¼ teaspoon black pepper
⅛ teaspoon cinnamon
2 tablespoons vegetable oil
½ bunch cilantro, washed and finely chopped
1 tablespoon minced garlic

Large skillet

Start to Finish
25 minutes
Serves 4

Preparation

• Thoroughly mix meat with salt, seven spices, pepper and cinnamon. Roll into 1-inch balls and set aside

Procedure

1• Place oil in a skillet over high heat, add meatballs, and sauté until brown.

2• Reduce heat to medium high, stir in cilantro and garlic, and sauté briefly. Add spinach, stir, and cook several more minutes.

3• Reduce heat to medium, adjust salt, and cook covered for 5 minutes. Remove from heat and serve.

Serve it hot with rice, plain yogurt and fresh pita bread.

** TIP Meat can be prepared a day in advance if refrigerated in a covered container.*

Nutrition Information per Serving

Calories 330, Fat 21g, Saturated fat 6g, Cholesterol 75mg, Carbohydrate 10g, Fiber 6g, Protein 29g

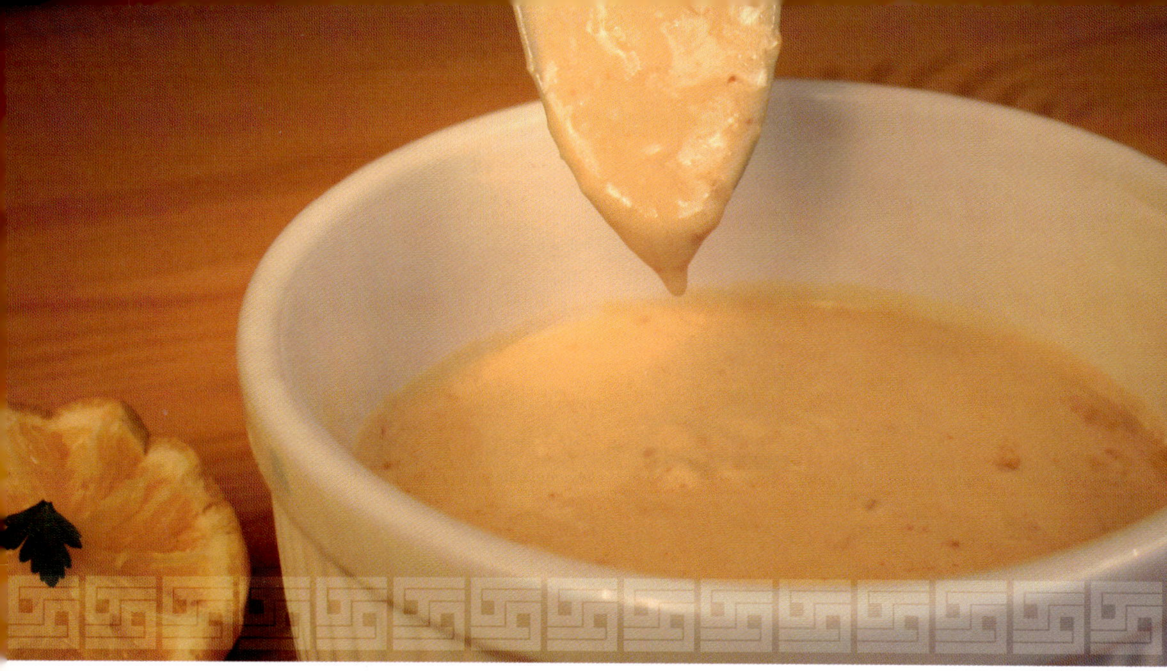

Tahini Sauce with Pine Nuts:

Salset Tahini b'Snoubar

صلصة طحينه بصنوبر

Ingredients

1 tablespoon olive oil
¼ cup pine nuts
⅓ cup tahini paste
1 teaspoon crushed garlic
1 cup water
¼ cup fresh lemon juice
¼ teaspoon salt

Slotted spoon
Paper towels
Electric food processor

Start to Finish
15 minutes

Procedure

1• Place oil in a small pot over medium-high heat, stir in pine nuts and sauté until golden brown. (Be careful, they burn easily.) With a slotted spoon, transfer nuts to a plate lined with paper towels and reserve oil.

2• Put tahini paste in a medium-sized bowl, stir in garlic and slowly add water while stirring in one direction until well mixed. Stir in lemon juice and salt, then pour the mixture into the pot with the reserved oil and place the pot over medium heat for 2 minutes.

3• Meanwhile, place drained pine nuts in the food processor, grind, and add to the mixture in the pot. Combine thoroughly and cook for 5 minutes, then turn off heat and serve.

Serve it hot or warm with fish and pita bread.

** TIP Tahini sauce can be mixed a couple of days in advance.*

Nutrition Information per Serving

Calories 128, Fat 12g, Saturated fat 1g, Cholesterol 0mg, Carbohydrate 4g, Fiber 1g, Protein 3g

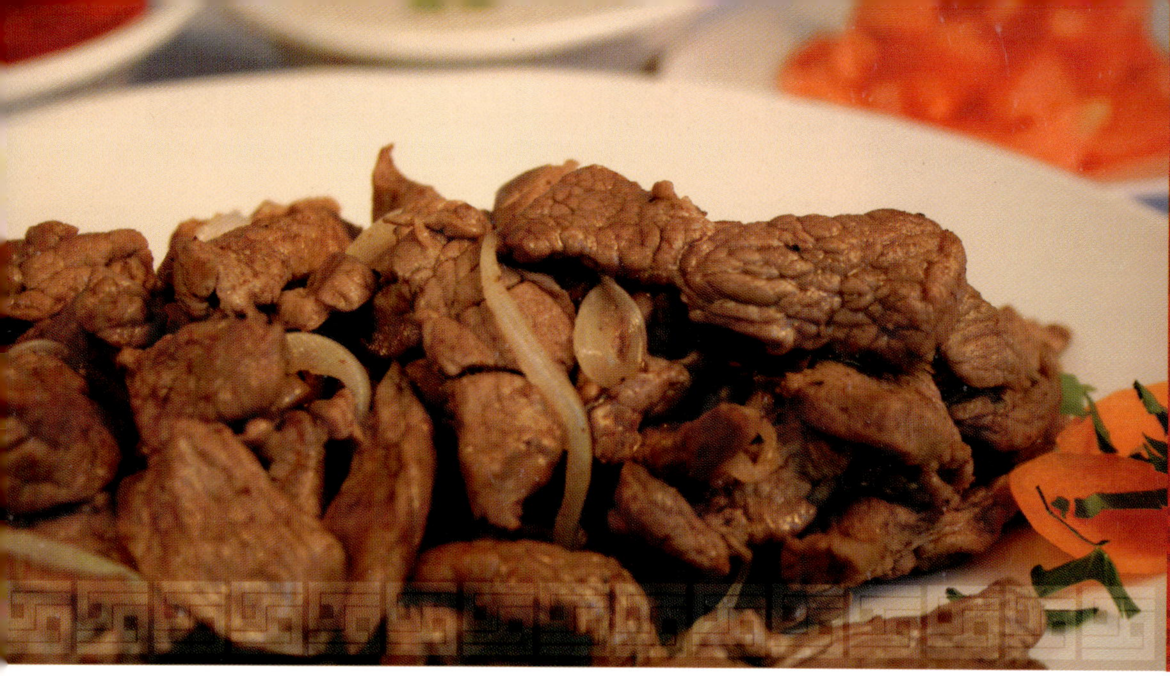

Top Sirloin Beef: Shawerma

شاورما

Ingredients

1½ pounds top sirloin beef, 1-inch thick
1 teaspoon salt
⅛ teaspoon ground black pepper,
¼ teaspoon ground seven spices
⅛ teaspoon ground cinnamon
¼ teaspoon cardamom
1¼ cups water
¼ cup vinegar

2 tablespoons butter or vegetable oil
1 small onion, thinly sliced (optional)
¼ teaspoon salt or to taste

Start to Finish
15 minutes
without marinating
Serves 4

Preparation

- Mix salt, black pepper, seven spices, cinnamon, water and vinegar in a bowl. Add meat to the mixture and set aside.
- Marinate overnight for best flavor.

Procedure

1• Drain marinated meat and cut it against the grain into strips that are ⅛-inch thick and about 2 inches wide.

2• Pour oil into a large pan and place over high heat. Add meat and sauté for 5 minutes or until brown.

3• Add onion and salt, sauté for another 5 minutes, and remove from heat.

Serve it with Tahini Sauce (see Vegetarian patties p:35), cucumber pickles, turnip pickles, thin tomato wedges, chopped parsley.

** TIP Shawerma makes a delicious sandwich.*

Nutrition Information per Serving

Calories 423, Fat 29g, Saturated fat 9g, Cholesterol 125mg, Carbohydrate 3.5g, Fiber 0g, Protein 42g

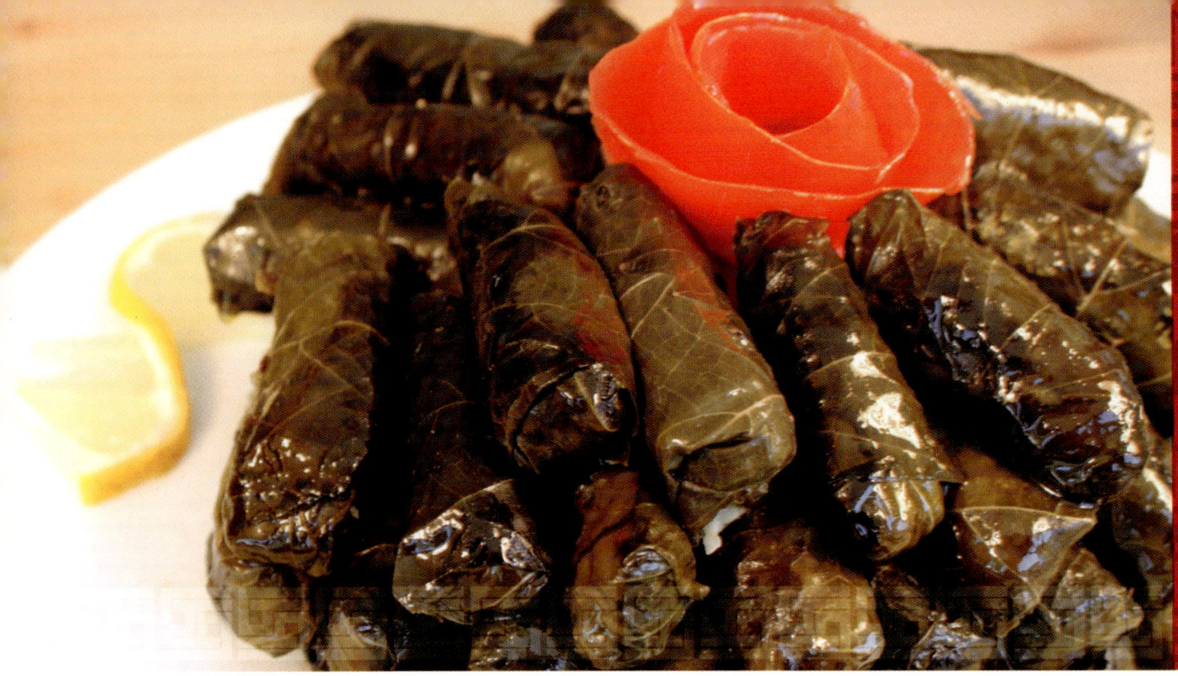

Vegetarian Grape Leaves: Warak Inab b'Zeit

ورق عنب بزيت

Ingredients

60 large preserved grape leaves (small jar)
1¼ cups short grain rice
½ cup parsley, finely chopped
½ cup mint leaves, finely chopped
1 cup peeled tomato, finely diced
½ cup diced onion
1 teaspoon salt or to taste
¼ teaspoon black pepper
½ cup fresh lemon juice
¼ cup olive oil

TO COOK:
Medium non-stick pot
2 medium potatoes
Salt and pepper to taste
2½ cups water
Heat-proof plate to fit in the pot

Start to Finish
1½ hours
Serves 6

Nutrition Information per Serving

Calories 423, Fat 29g, Saturated fat 9g, Cholesterol 125mg, Carbohydrate 3.5g, Fiber 0g, Protein 42g

Preparation

• Rinse preserved grape leaves with water until the water runs clear, drain, trim stems off the leaves and set aside.
• FILLING: Rinse and drain parsley, then cut off most of the stalk and discard. Chop it finely, measure and place in a large bowl.
• Rinse and drain mint leaves, chop finely and measure, then place in bowl over parsley. Peel onion, chop finely, measure and place over mint. Peel and dice tomato, measure, and place in bowl over onion.
• Rinse and drain rice, then place in bowl over the chopped vegetables. Add salt, pepper, lemon juice and olive oil, mix well and set aside.

Procedure

1• On a working surface, spread 5 grape leaves at a time, with the shiny side down and the trimmed stem close to you. Spoon 1 tablespoon filling and place it near the trimmed end in a thin row across the width of the leaf.

2• Fold the stem end over to partly enclose the filling, then fold the sides over it and roll firmly from stem to tip.

3• Finish remaining leaves in the same way and reserve filling sauce.

4• Wash and peel potatoes, and cut into ¼-inch slices. Coat the pot with olive oil and layer sliced potatoes at the bottom. Place stuffed leaves in tight rows to cover the potatoes, with the loose sides down. Place additional layers of rows until all the stuffed leaves are in the pot.

5• Sprinkle with salt and pepper, and slowly pour in reserved sauce.

6• Invert a heavy, heat-proof plate and place it over the rolled leaves to hold them in place while cooking. (Make sure the plate is ¼ inch smaller then the pot). Slowly pour in 2¼ cups water and bring to a boil over high heat for 5 minutes. Reduce heat to medium and cook for 30 more minutes. Reduce again heat to low and cook for another 20 minutes. Turn off heat and let the pot sit, untouched, for another half hour. Remove the plate, then invert a serving platter and place it over the pot. Hold both platter and pot tightly and slowly invert both, let stuffed grape leaves slide to the platter, and then gently remove the pot.

Serve it warm or cold as an appetizer.

** TIP This meal can be prepared and cooked 5 days in advance*

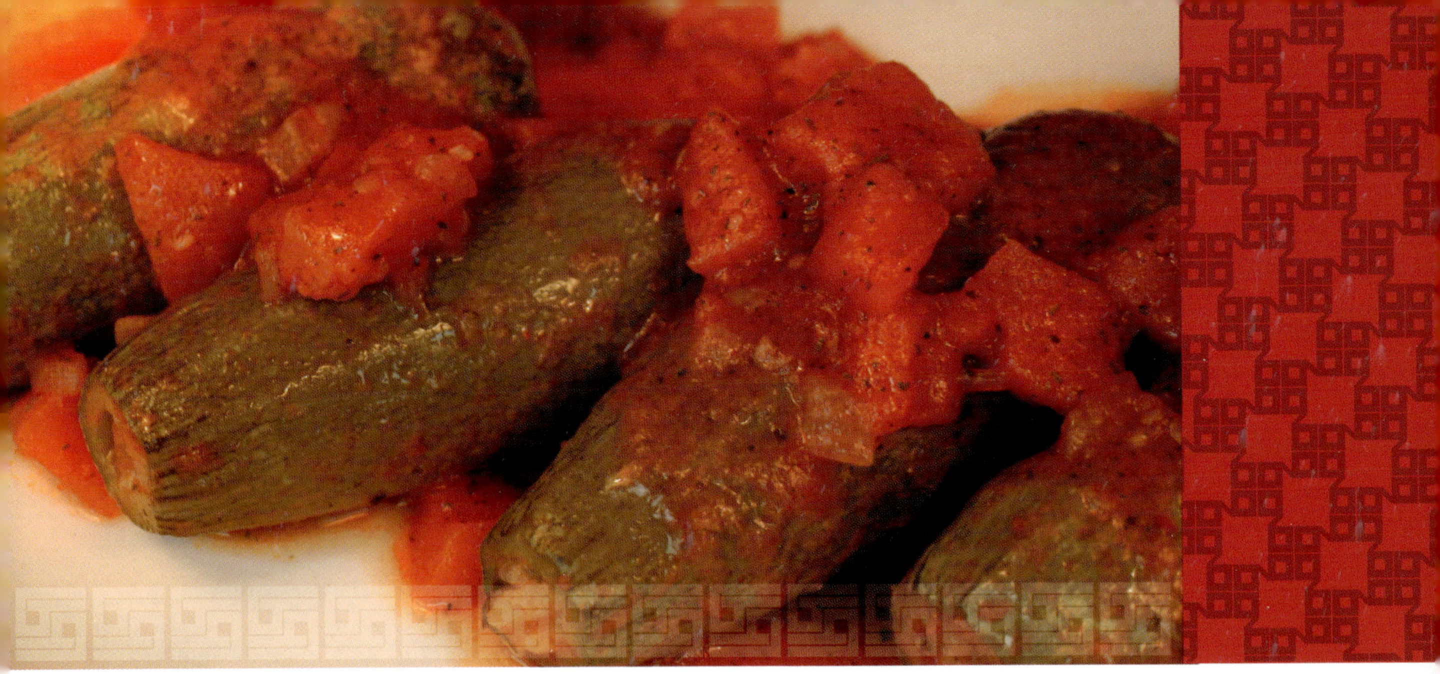

Stuffed meals (Mahashi المحاشي) are at the heart of authentic Lebanese cuisine. There are three types of traditional fillings for stuffed meals: vegetarian, consisting of rice, tomatoes, onion, herbs, and spices; ground meat with rice and spices; and meat and spices with pine nuts. Once they are stuffed, the vegetables are cooked in either tomato sauce, a mixture of crushed garlic, dried mint and lemon juice, or simply in lemon juice and water. I have worked very hard to simplify this recipe. It still takes over half an hour to prepare and cook a stuffed meal, but I'm sure you'll agree that the end result is worth the time and effort.

This meal is a favorite meal of my daughters Nadine and Ashly

Vegetarian Stuffed Squash:

Kousa Mahshi b'Zeit

كوسا محشي بزيت

Ingredients

12 medium summer squash, cored
1 cup short grain rice, washed and drained
½ cup chopped fresh parsley
½ cup tomato, finely diced
¼ cup chopped fresh mint
¼ cup chopped onion
½ teaspoon salt
⅛ teaspoon black pepper
¼ cup fresh lemon juice
2 tablespoons olive oil

To Cook

2 tablespoons olive oil
1 cup tomatoes, peeled and diced
½ teaspoon sugar
1 cup tomato sauce
½ teaspoon salt or to taste
4 cups water
2 teaspoons dry mint
2 teaspoons crushed garlic

Preparation

- Cored squash prepared and set aside
- Large pot

Coring the squash P. 130

Start to Finish
40 minutes
plus cored zucchini
Serves 4

Nutrition Information per Serving

Calories 386, Fat 14g, Saturated fat 2g, Cholesterol 0mg, Carbohydrate 59g, Fiber 5g, Protein 8g

Procedure

1• Place rice, parsley, tomatoes, mint, onion, salt, pepper, lemon juice and oil in a medium-sized bowl and mix well.

2• Place 2 tablespoons olive oil in a large pot over medium heat and add diced tomato and sugar. Cook for 7 minutes while you are filling the squash, then add tomato sauce, salt and water, stir, and bring to a boil over high heat.

3• Meanwhile, hold one cored squash in your left hand, pick up some filling with your right hand and feed it through the opening, leaving ½ inch empty at the top. To make sure that the squash is well filled, hold the squash with the opening at the top, place your thumb over the opening, and shake the squash several times in a downward motion. Look through the opening to determine if it needs more filling.

4• Finish the remaining squash in the same way and gently place them inside the boiling pot. Strain the seasoned tomato sauce over it and let it cook for 5 minutes, then reduce heat to medium and cook covered for 20 minutes.

5• Uncover the pot, sprinkle mint, add garlic, and gently stir to blend. Cover and simmer for 5 more minutes or until the rice is soft, then turn off the heat and let it sit for few minutes. Transfer to a deep platter and serve.

Serve it hot or warm with fresh pita bread, green pepper and Arugula and Watercress Salad.

** TIP Squash can be cored and stuffed a couple of days in advance and stored in a covered container in the refrigerator. You can even stuff green peppers, tomatoes, grape leaves and small eggplants, and cook them together.*

Coring the squash: Na'ar L'Kousa

Ingredients

12 fresh squash at room temperature

squash corer

Start to Finish
15 minutes

Procedure

1• Wash and drain squash. With a sharp knife, discard stem end and shave off the bottom brown skins.

2• Place squash in the palm of your left hand (if you're right handed, and the opposite if you're left handed) with the cut top facing you. Cup your fingers around it and hold firmly while you are slowly inserting the corer into the middle top half way down inside the squash. Twirl the corer clock wise inside the squash to loosen the pulp, and then pull the corer out slowly. With your finger slide the squash pulp off the corer onto a plate, then insert the corer back inside the squash to remove as much pulp as possible, with a circular motion from the sides and the bottom, leaving 1/8-inch thick wall, then set-aside in a large bowl.

3• Finish coring the remaining squash. Wash them inside and out with cold water and drain, ready to use.

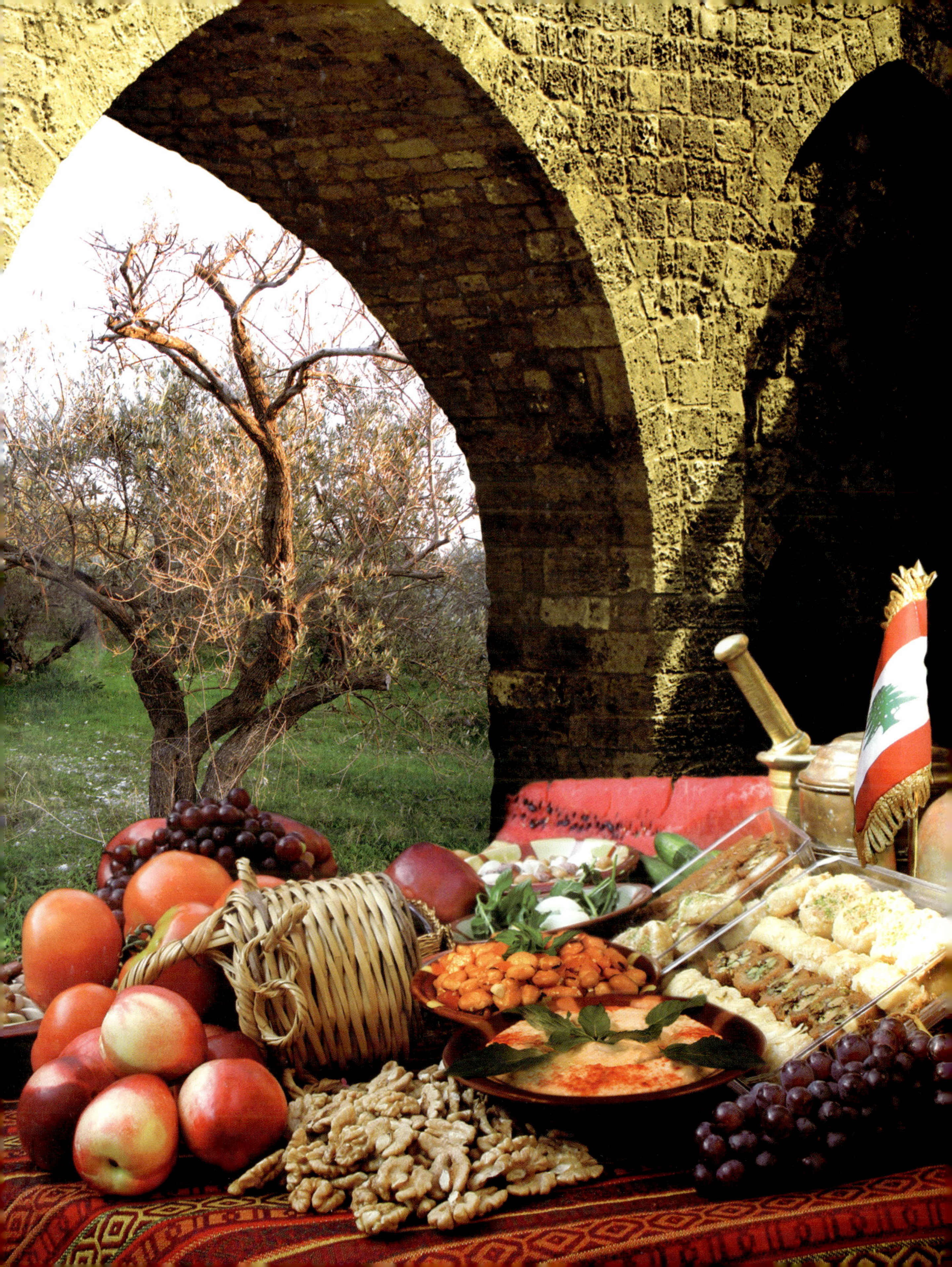

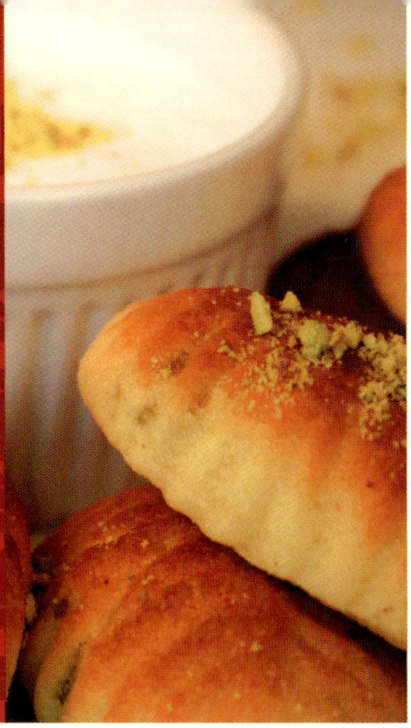
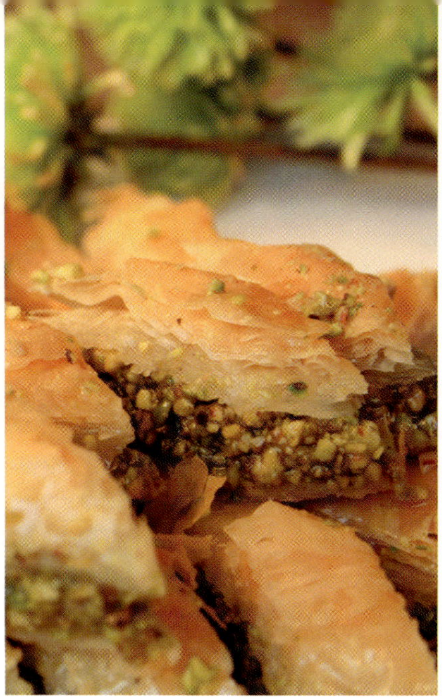
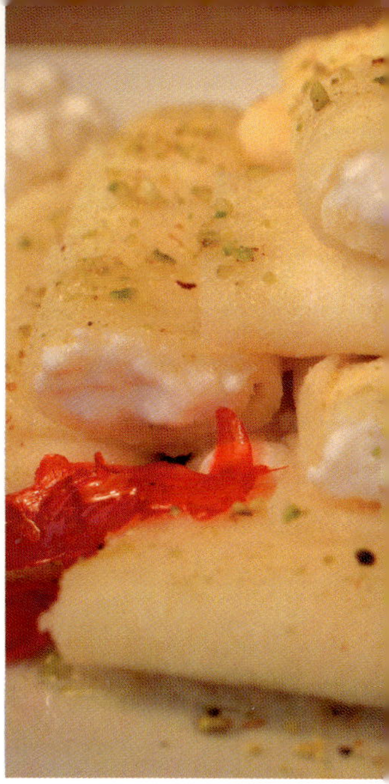

Sweets: El Halaweyat

الحلويات

Tripoli (North of Lebanon) has long been celebrated for its sweets (Halaweyat). It is famous for making cream-filled cheese fingers Halawet al jiben and nutty sweets like Baklawa that are available year-round. Buses and vehicles line up daily in front of the well-known shops in Tripoli for people to buy their favorite delicacies before leaving on a trip. Some sweets are enjoyed in the morning as breakfast like K'nafee b'kaak, a national favorite. My father used to leave early in the morning to buy k'nafee for us before we went to school. Sweets are also served in the afternoon after a nap or at a big gatherings or parties.

Cakes and puddings are delicious treats for family and friends and, as we all know, they are appropriate at most any time of the day.

Holiday treats (Halaweyat lil A'yad wal Moonasabet) are available in the shops only during the holidays or by placing an order. But preparing your own holiday treats at home adds to the excitement of the season, and fills the house with familiar and tempting aromas. My mother spent hours fixing the holiday treats (Ma'mool) for our family of 10, and she always had extra on hand when relatives and guests came to visit. She wisely baked some treats at home and sent the rest in large, round pans to a bakery to be cooked, saving her time and effort.

Mainly the dessert could be anything from the above or fresh fruits of your choice or even dry fruit like figs or dates and in this chapter you will find many choices to delight your taste buds!

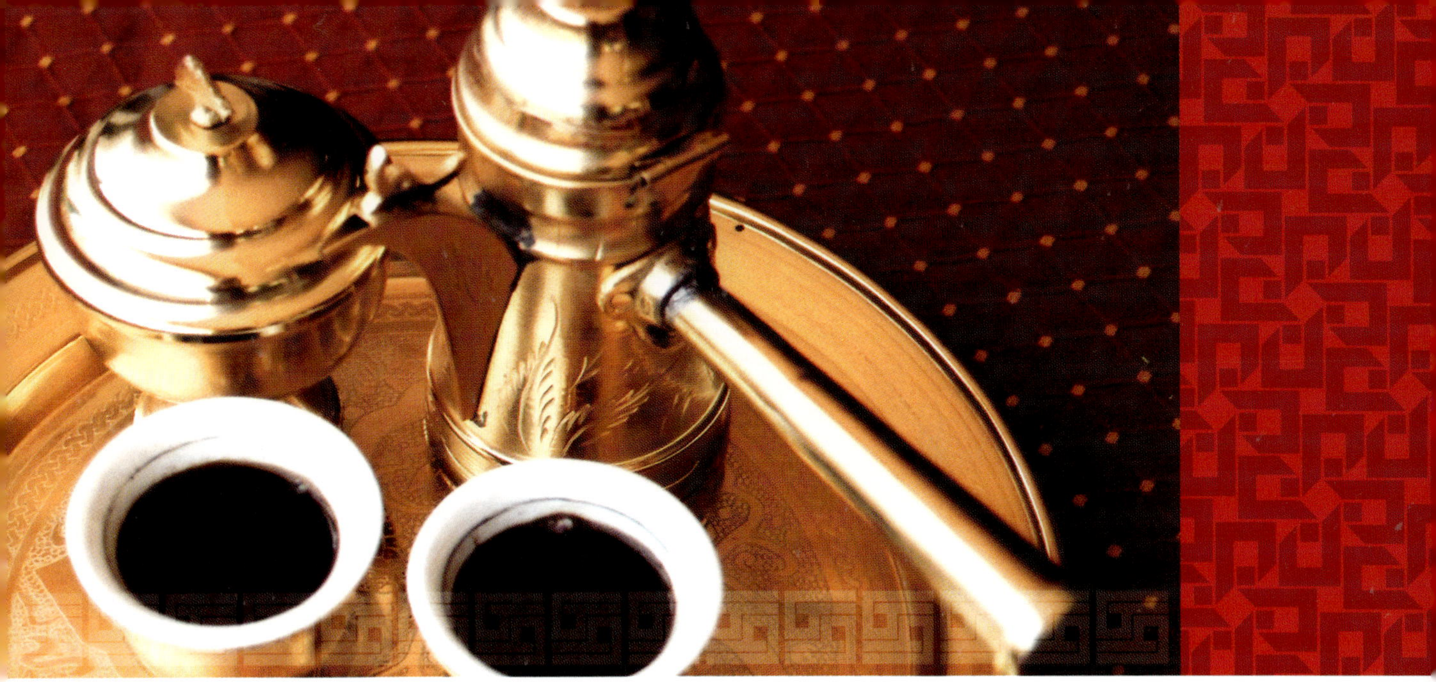

In Lebanon, coffee drinkers gather on balconies and verandahs before breakfast in towns and villages throughout the country, and homemakers prepare a rakweh or pot of coffee to take to their neighbor's for the subhiyeh, the morning chat. Coffee is consumed after lunch, during the evening and throughout the working day. All day you can see and hear the coffee sellers plying their wares to workmen in the city. After drinking your coffee, you may be fortunate enough to find yourself with someone who will be able to predict your future by the patterns left by your coffee grinds. (I was lucky because my neighbor used to predict my future and I loved it!) Coffee is served at important meetings and funerals but never at weddings, where more fitting beverages are produced.

Arabic Coffee: Kahweh Arabi

قهوة عربي

Ingredients

¾ cup water
¼ teaspoon sugar or to taste
3 teaspoons ground Arabic coffee

Small coffee pot (rakweh)
Small coffee cups or domed cups

Start to Finish
7 minutes
Serves 3

Procedure

1• Pour water into the coffee pot and bring to a boil over high heat.

2• Reduce heat to low and add sugar, if desired. Stir in coffee and heat until just before it boils.

3• Turn off heat and set coffee aside to settle for a few seconds, then slowly pour it into the cups and serve.

Serve it hot with a glass of water and cookies of your choice.

** TIP Arabic coffee, rakweh, and domed cups can be found in any Middle Eastern store or international market. Ask for a Turkish grind, choose the blend and they will grind it fresh for you. My own blend is half dark-half light roasting beans with a bit of ground cardamom. If you prefer the coffee stronger, just add more ground coffee to the boiling water.*

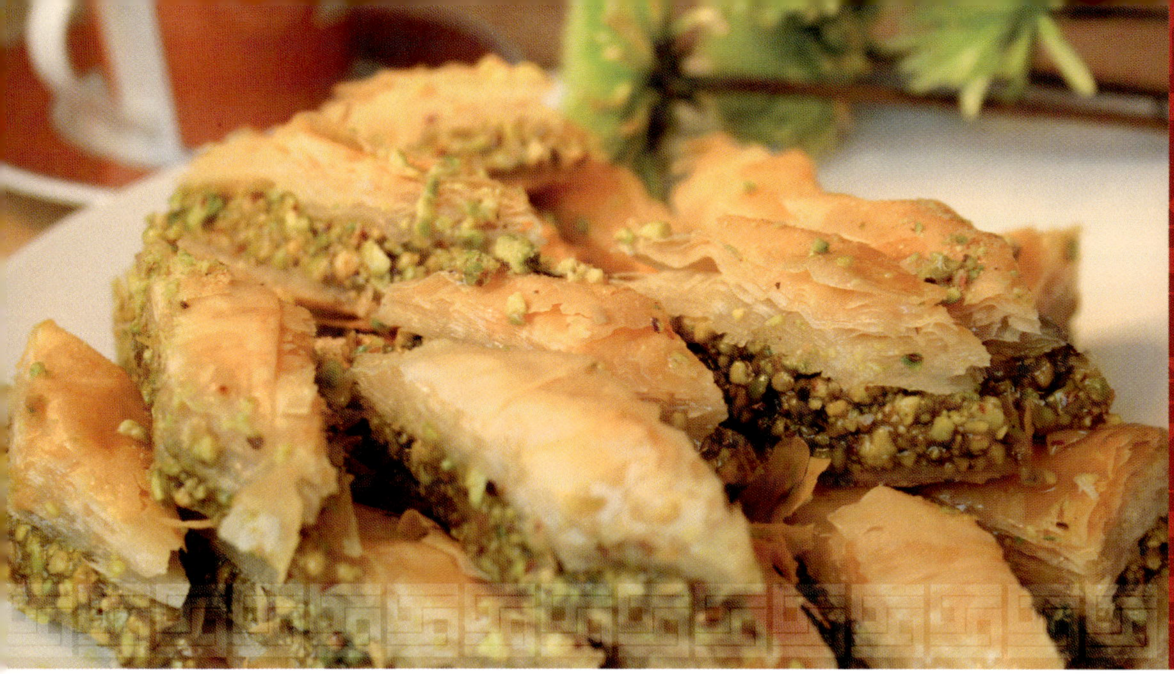

Baklava: Baklawa

بقلاوة

Ingredients

1 recipe Lebanese Syrup at room temperature
16 ounces phyllo dough at room temperature
¾ pound raw pistachio nuts
⅓ cup sugar
2 tablespoons rose water
¾ cup melted clarified butter

Electric food processor
12 x 9 x 2-inch greased pan
Pastry brush

Start to finish
20 minutes
plus syrup recipe
and baking time
Serves 12

Procedure

1• Preheat oven to 375 degrees F.

2• Place pistachio nuts in the food processor and process until finely crushed. Reserve 2 tablespoons for garnish. In a bowl, combine remaining crushed nuts with sugar. Add rose water and stir until thoroughly moistened.

3• Carefully unroll phyllo sheets onto a smooth, dry surface and cut them in half. Cover immediately with plastic wrap and then with a damp towel. Place melted butter, greased pan and pastry brush next to phyllo sheets.

4• Remove 4 phyllo sheets, place them in the greased pan and promptly recover the others. Dip pastry brush in the melted butter and brush the entire surface of the top sheet; top these with another 4 phyllo sheets and brush in the same way, then add 4 more sheets and brush the top again.

5• Now, place 4 phyllo sheets on each side of the pan, with half of the sheets resting inside the pan, and the remaining half of the sheets outside of the pan.
Brush the entire surface with butter.

6• Add 4 more sheets and spread pistachio mixture over the entire surface. Gently press mixture with your fingertips to insure an even thickness throughout the pan. Flip all the sides of the phyllo resting on the outside over the pistachio to cover and then brush with butter.

7• Continue to add 4 phyllo sheets at a time, brushing the top sheet with butter, until only 4 remain. With a dull knife, finish the brushed sheets by tucking edges down the sides of the pan. Add 3 of the remaining sheets, brush top and sides with butter, then add the last sheet. With a sharp knife, gently cut through all layers to form triangles, diamonds or shape of your choice; gently brush with clarified butter to moisten and seal edges.

8• Bake for 30 minutes or until golden brown. Remove pan from oven and promptly pour Lebanese syrup evenly over baklava, garnish with crushed nuts and set aside to cool.

Serve at room temperature for dessert.

** TIP Baklava stays fresh up to 2 weeks if cooled and then kept in a covered container.*

Nutrition Information per Serving

Calories 334, Fat 22g, Saturated fat 9g, Cholesterol 35mg, Carbohydrate 29g, Fiber 2g, Protein 5g

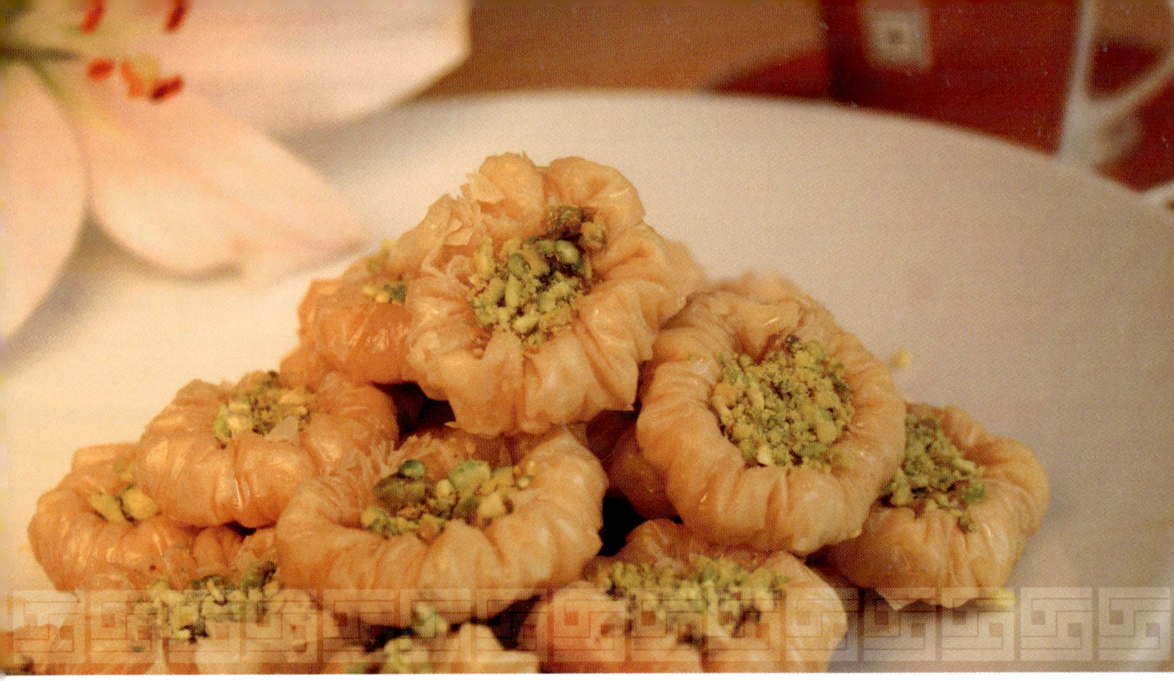

Bird's Nest with Pistachio Nuts:

A'sh el Bolbol

عش البلبل

Ingredients

1 recipe Lebanese Syrup
Phyllo dough at room temperature (follow Instructions on the box)
2 cups finely crushed pistachio nuts
3 tablespoons sugar
1½ tablespoons rose water
½ cup melted clarified butter

Pastry brush
18-inch dowel that is ¼ inch thick
Greased 16- x11-inch pan or to fit

Start to finish
20 minutes
plus syrup recipe
and baking time
Serves 30

Preparation

Lebanese Syrup prepared and set aside at room temperature

Procedure

1• Preheat oven to 350 degrees F.

2• Measure 1½ cups pistachio nuts and place in a bowl. Add sugar, stir to combine, then add rose water and mix until moistened. Set nut mixture on working counter with melted butter, pastry brush and dowel. Reserve remaining 1/2 cup of crushed nuts for a garnish.

3• Carefully unroll phyllo sheets onto a smooth, dry surface beside you and follow instructions on the box.

4• Remove one phyllo sheet and promptly recover the others. Place phyllo sheet on the counter and line up the dowel in the middle of the bottom half of the sheet. Fold the bottom fourth of the phyllo over the dowel up to the middle of the sheet. Sprinkle 1 teaspoon or more of the nut mixture in a thin row by the dowel and roll firmly, leaving 1 inch at the tip of the sheet unrolled. Hold the dowel at the ends with two hands and push both sides of the rolled sheet to the middle, forming a fringe with the dough.

5• Gently slide the fringe off the dowel. Gather the two ends with the loose 1-inch tip in the middle, creating a circle that looks like a nest.

6• Place nest in the pan and finish the remaining sheets in the same way. Gently brush with clarified butter until covered, and place pan in the oven to bake until dough nests are golden brown.

7• Once they are out of the oven hot, gently pour syrup over the nests. Fill the middle of each nest with 1 teaspoon of the remaining crushed pistachio nuts, set aside to cool and then serve.

Serve at room temperature for dessert.

** TIP Bird's Nest stays fresh up to a month if kept in a covered container after cooling. Vegetable oil may be used in place of clarified butter. Recipe can be split in half.*

Nutrition Information per Serving

Calories 107, Fat 5g, Saturated fat 1g, Cholesterol 3mg, Carbohydrate 15g, Fiber 1g, Protein 2g

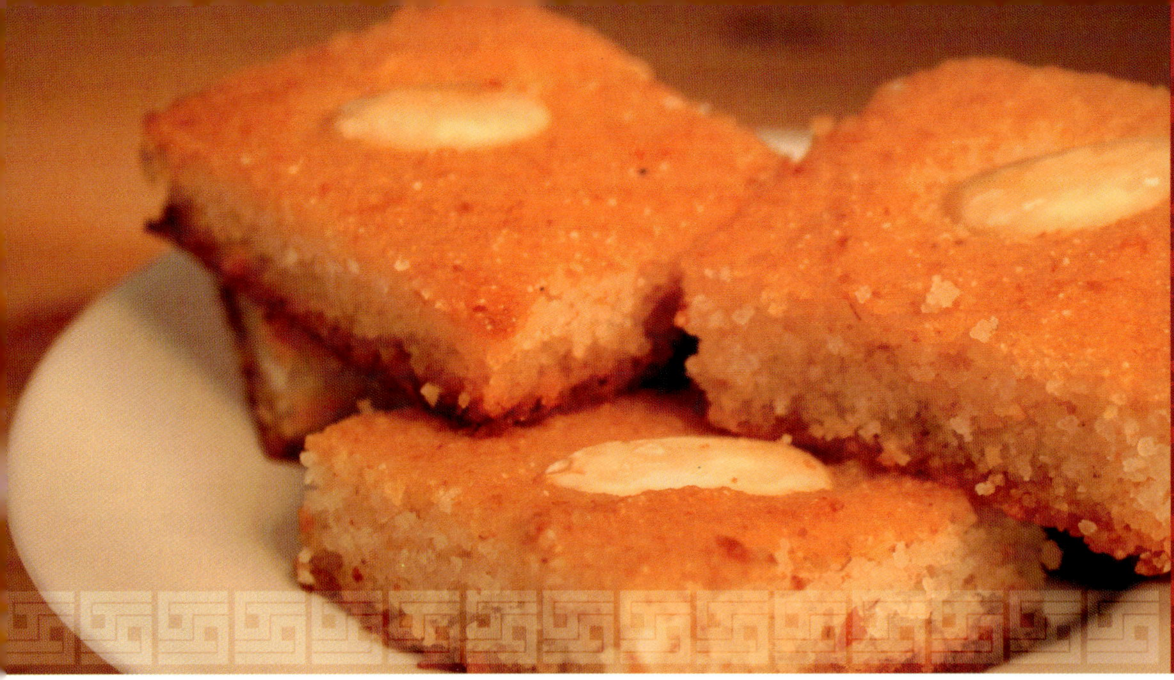

Cream of Wheat Cake: Namoorah

نمورة

Ingredients

1 recipe Lebanese Syrup
½ cup butter
¾ cup milk
1¼ cups plain yogurt
1 tablespoon orange blossom water
2 cups farina
1 cup granulated sugar
¼ teaspoon baking soda
¼ cup blanched almonds, sliced
2 tablespoon finely crushed pistachio nuts to garnish

Start to Finish
10 minutes
plus syrup preparation and baking
time Serves 12

Heat oven to 375 degrees F.
12 ¼"x 8 x 1.5 inch pan
1 tablespoon tahini sauce

Preparation

• Prepare Lebanese Syrup recipe a day in advance, if possible. The syrup should be at room temperature.

Procedure

1• Heat oven to 375 degrees F.

2• Pour milk into a medium-sized saucepan, and add butter, yogurt and orange blossom water. Place pan over medium heat until butter melts.

3• In a large bowl, combine semolina, sugar, and baking soda.

4• Coat bottom and sides of baking pan with tahini sauce and set aside.

5• Pour butter mixture over dry mixture and stir with a spoon until well mixed.

6• Pour batter into the tahini-coated pan. Tap the pan on the counter top several times to make the surface smooth and even.

7• Gently place almonds (25 pieces) on the surface 1½ inches apart from each other.

8• Bake for 30 minutes or until golden brown.

9• Remove from oven and immediately pour syrup evenly over the surface. Sprinkle pistachio nuts over the syrup and set aside to cool.

10• Square it with a sharp knife and serve at room temperature.

Serve for dessert or as a snack.

** TIP ½ cup finely shredded dried coconut can be added to the batter.*

Nutrition Information per Serving

Calories 278, Fat 8g, Saturated fat 3g, Cholesterol 14mg, Carbohydrate 49g, Fiber 1g, Protein 4g

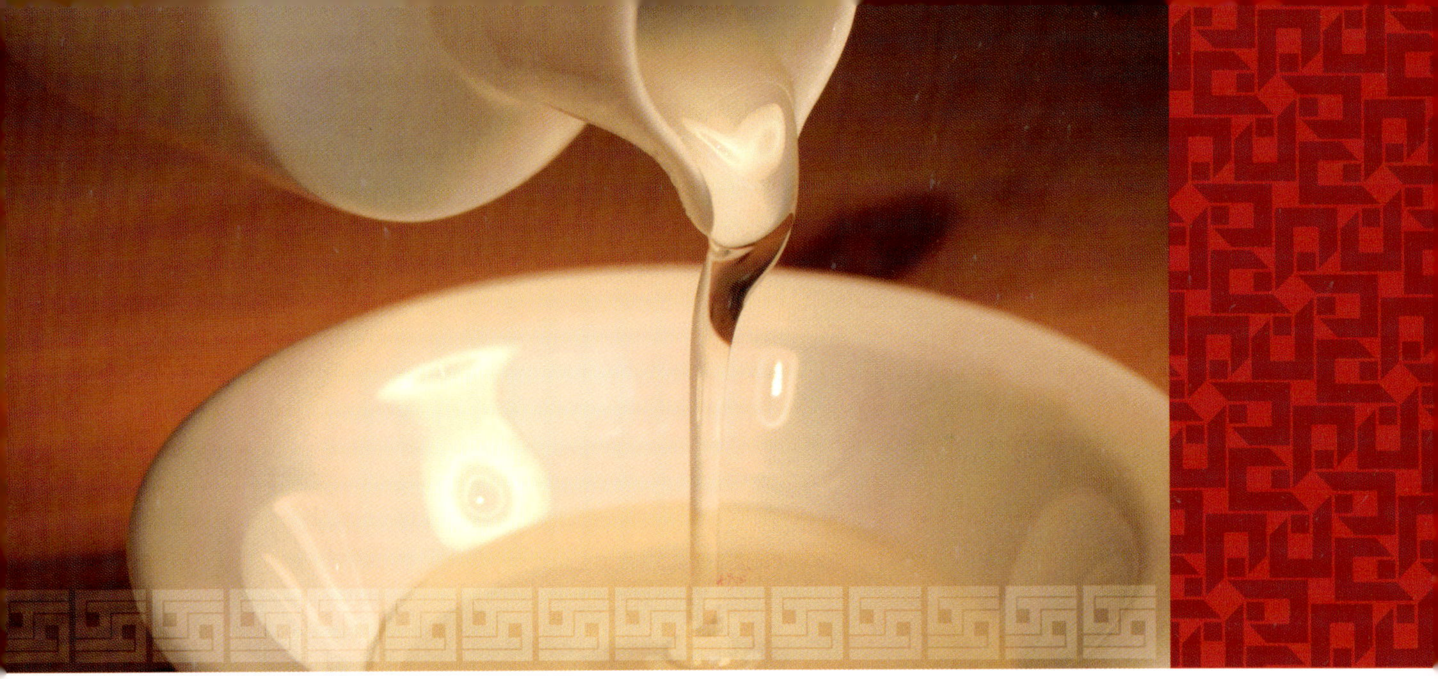

Lebanese Syrup: Katter

قطر

Ingredients

2 cups granulated sugar
1 cup water
1 teaspoon lemon juice
1 teaspoon rose water

Start to Finish
15 minutes

Nutrition Information per Serving

Calories 81, Fat 0g, Saturated fat 0g, Cholesterol 0mg, Carbohydrate 21g, Fiber 0g, Protein 0g

Procedure

1• In a medium saucepan, mix sugar and water with a wooden spoon and place on the stove over high heat. Bring to boil for 7 minutes, stirring occasionally.

2• Reduce heat to medium-high, cover and cook for several minutes. Remove cover, stir in lemon juice and cook for 2 more minutes; add rose water, stir well, turn off heat and set aside to cool.

Serve it with sweets that call for syrup.

** TIP Lebanese Syrup can be made a week in advance.*

Holiday Pastry Dough: Ajeennit l'Ma'mool

عجينة المعمول

Ingredients

1 teaspoon active yeast
1 teaspoon sugar
¼ cup warm water
2 cups fine semolina
1 cup all-purpose flour
1 teaspoon ground mahlab
3 tablespoons sugar
1 cup unsalted butter
½ cup milk
3 tablespoons orange blossom water

Start to Finish
10 minutes

Nutrition Information per Serving

Calories 60, Fat 2g, Saturated fat 1g, Cholesterol 5mg, Carbohydrate 9g, Fiber 0g, Protein 1g

Procedure

1• In a cup, combine yeast, sugar and water, and set aside.

2• In a large bowl, combine semolina, flour, mahlab and sugar, and set it aside.

3• Put butter in a small saucepan; add milk and place over medium heat until the butter melts.

4• Pour milk and butter mixture into the semolina bowl and mix well. Add yeast mixture and orange blossom water, mix again to combine, then cover with plastic wrap and set aside.

** TIP The dough can be made a day in advance and refrigerated. Return dough to room temperature before you use it.*

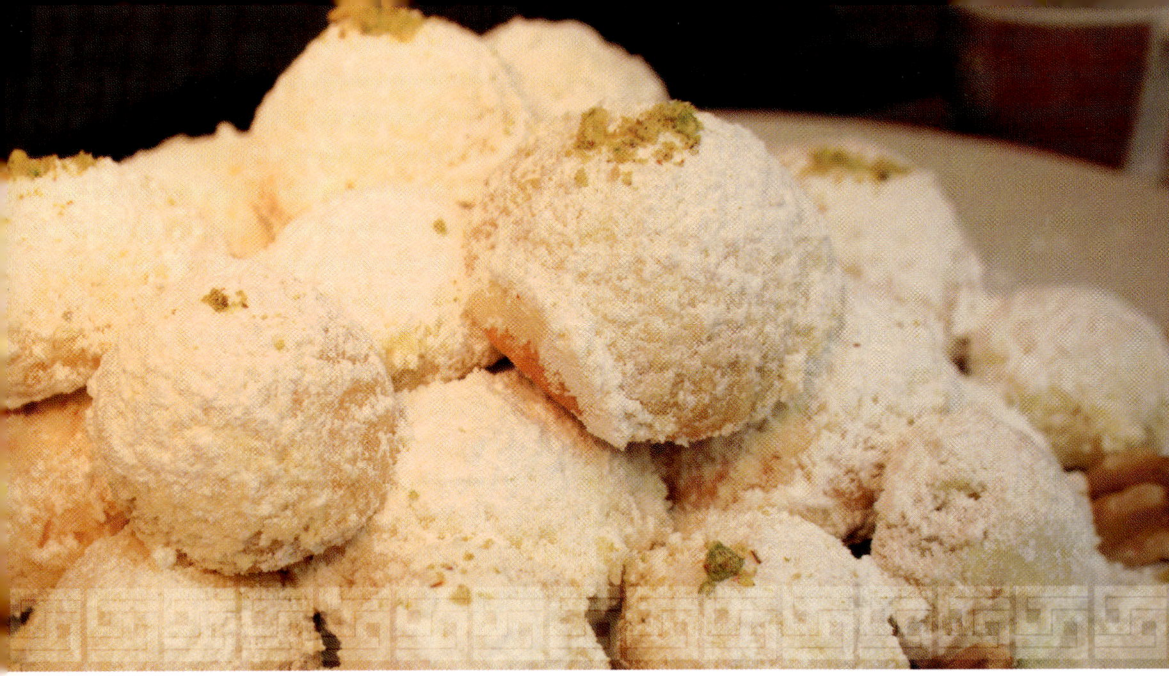

Walnut-filled Pastry: Ma'mool b'Joz

معمول بجوز

Ingredients

1 recipe Holiday Pastry Dough
2 cups coarsely crushed walnuts
½ cup sugar
1½ tablespoons rose water
Ma'mool mold

17x12-inch pan or any pan to fit
1 cup powdered sugar
Sifter

Start to Finish
30 minutes
plus dough recipe
and baking time
Makes about
35 pieces

Preparation

- Holiday Pastry Dough prepared and set aside.
- Place chopped walnuts in a medium-sized bowl. Add sugar and mix well to combine.
- Drizzle rose water over the walnut mixture while stirring until the mixture is wet, then set aside.

Procedure

1• Heat oven to 375 degrees F.

2• Take a small piece of the dough, a bit bigger then a walnut, in the palm of your hand, and flatten it with your fingers into a circle ⅛ inch thick.

3• Place 1 tablespoon filling in the center of the dough circle and press it with your thumb. Bring up the sides of the dough to cover the filling and close. It should be a firm ball that you can roll between the palms of your hands.

4• Put the ball in a Ma'mool mold, press gently to flatten and smooth the top surface. Turn mold upside down with one hand; tap the mold on the edge of the counter to loosen the pastry while holding the other hand under the mold to catch it.

5• Place pastry in the pan; repeat with the remaining dough and filling until they are all gone. If mold is not available, shape pastry into a dome and decorate by pressing fork prongs around the top. Or, ask your children and they will come up with some very creative shapes!

6• Bake in preheated oven for 30 minutes or until they turn golden in color. Remove from oven and set aside.

7• Put the powdered sugar in a sifter and sprinkle over the top of the hot pastry.

8• Let it cool to room temperature and store it in a covered container for up to 2 weeks.

Serve at room temperature around the holidays or anytime for dessert.

** TIP Ma'mool mold is a wooden dome that is slightly pointed and deeply carved on the inside; it is used to form and decorate holiday pastries. It is about 3 inches in diameter with a thick handle and can be found in any Middle Eastern market.*

Nutrition Information per Serving

Calories 123, Fat 7g, Saturated fat 2g, Cholesterol 5mg, Carbohydrate 14g, Fiber 1g, Protein 2g

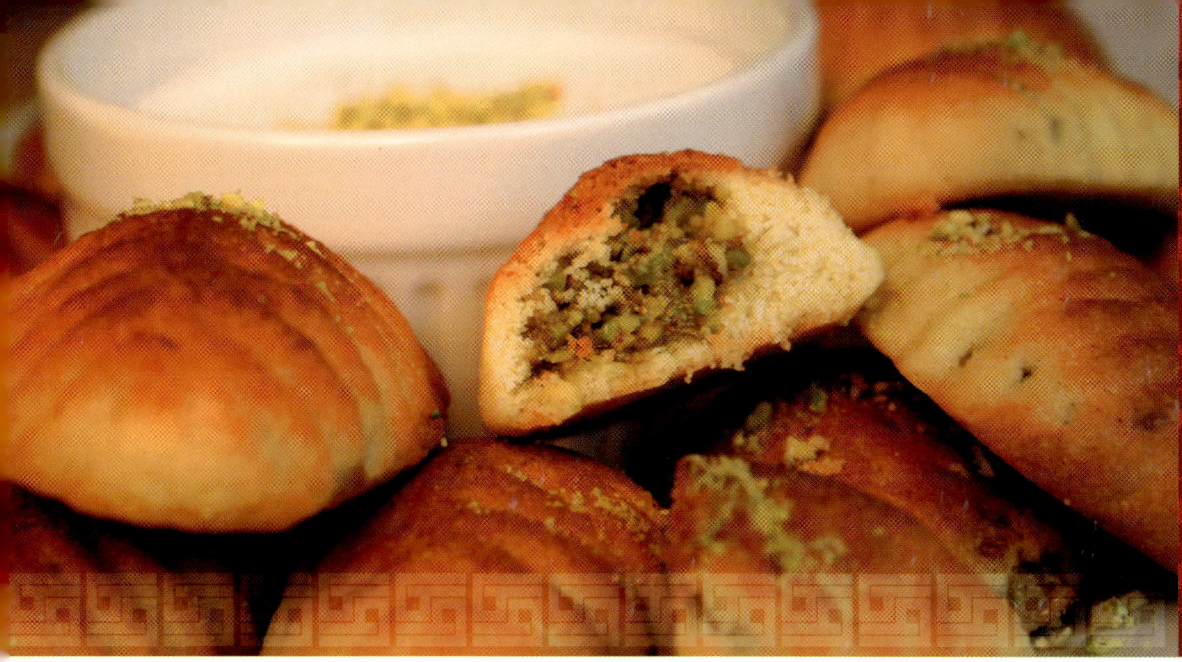

Pistachio-filled Pastry: Karbouj Halab

كربوج حلب

Ingredients

1 teaspoon yeast
¼ cup warm water
3 cups fine semolina
1 teaspoon mahlab
1 cup unsalted butter
½ cup milk
1 tablespoon orange blossom water

Karbouj halab Mold*
9x12-inch pan
TOPPING:
One 8-ounce jar marshmallow creme
1 tablespoon rose water

Nutrition Information per Serving

Calories 115, Fat 5g, Saturated fat 2g, Cholesterol 5mg, Carbohydrate 14g, Fiber 1g, Protein 3g

PISTACHIO FILLING: Hashwit Fistok

- 2 cups coarsely crushed pistachio nuts
- ½ cup sugar
- 2 tablespoons rose water

In a bowl, combine sugar and pistachio nuts, drizzle with rose water and mix well to combine. The mixture should be a bit wet.

Start to Finish
30 minutes
plus baking time
Makes 35 pieces

Preparation

• In a cup, combine yeast, sugar and water, set aside for several minutes.
• Combine semolina and mahlab and set aside. Put butter and milk in a small saucepan over medium heat until the butter melts, and then pour it over the semolina mixture. Add orange blossom water and mix well to combine. Cover with plastic wrap and set aside for 5 minutes.
• In the meantime, prepare Pistachio Filling and set aside.

Procedure

1• Preheat oven to 375 degrees F.

2• Take a small amount of semolina dough, a bit larger than a walnut, in the palm of your hand. Flatten the dough with your other hand into a circle ⅛ inch thick.

3• Place 1 tablespoon filling in the center of dough circle and press dough and filling flat with your thumb. Bring up the sides of the dough to cover the filling and close it. Roll the ball between the palms of your hands until it is smooth.

4• Put the filled dough in the Karbouj halab mold, press gently to flatten and smooth the top surface. Turn mold upside down with one hand; tap the mold on the edge of the counter to loosen the pastry while holding the other hand under the mold to catch it.

5• Place pastry in the pan; repeat with the remaining dough and filling until they are all gone. Bake for 30 minutes or until they turn golden in color.

6• Meanwhile, open jar of marshmallow crème and place it in the microwave for 10 seconds. Add 1 tablespoon rose water and mix well to combine.

7• When pastries are done and still hot, pour marshmallow topping to cover all the pastries or serve it separately by dipping the pastry in the marshmallow.

Serve at room temperature around the holidays or for dessert or a snack anytime.

**TIP Karbouj Halab mold is oval in shape. It measures about 3 inches in diameter and has a thick handle. It can be found at any Middle Eastern store.*

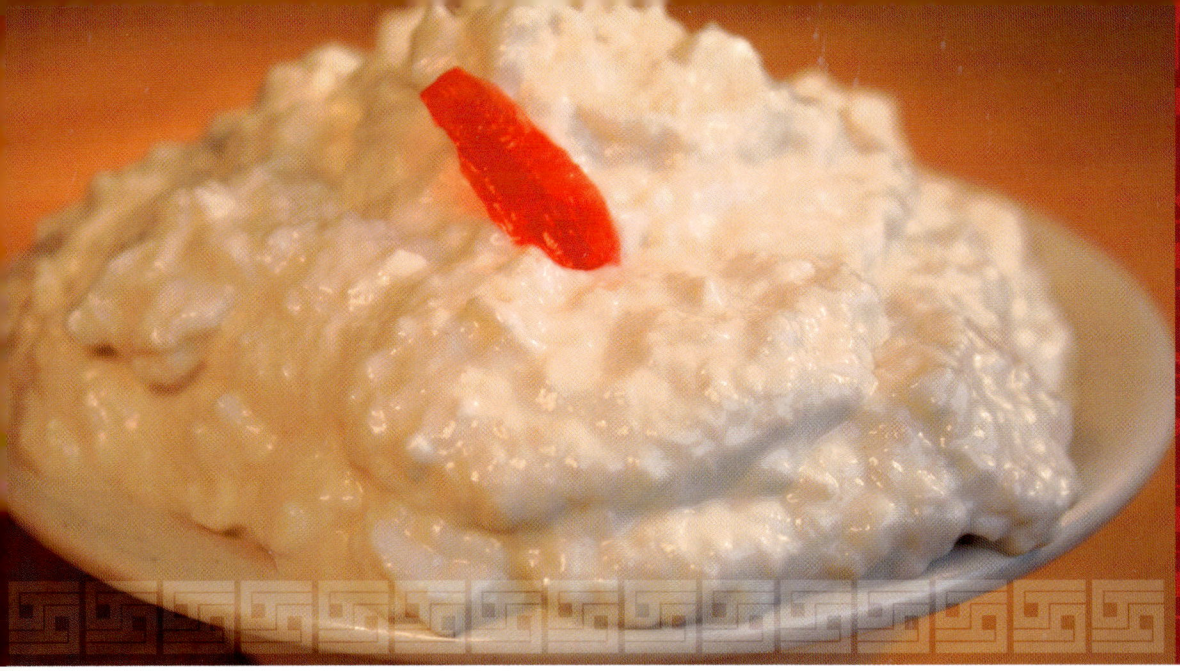

Clotted Cream: Kashtah

قشطه

Ingredients

1 quart half-and-half
¼ cup cornstarch
8 slices white bread
2 tablespoon granulated sugar
1 tablespoon orange blossom water

Start to finish
15 minutes

Preparation

Cut off crust and discard. Break bread into small pieces and set aside

Procedure

1• Pour ½ cup half-and-half into a medium-sized pot, add cornstarch and stir until it dissolves. Pour in remaining half-and-half and stir well to combine.

2• Add bread pieces and mix thoroughly.

3• Place pot over medium-high heat, add sugar and continue to stir slowly in one direction until mixture thickens and starts to bubble.

4• Reduce heat to low, add 1 tablespoon rose water, and stir for another minute. Turn off heat and set aside to cool.

Serve it cold or at room temperature as a filling or by itself with honey for breakfast.

** TIP Clotted Cream can be refrigerated up to a week.*

Nutrition Information per Serving

Calories 95, Fat 6g, Saturated fat 3.5g, Cholesterol 18mg, Carbohydrate 9g, Fiber 0g, Protein 2g

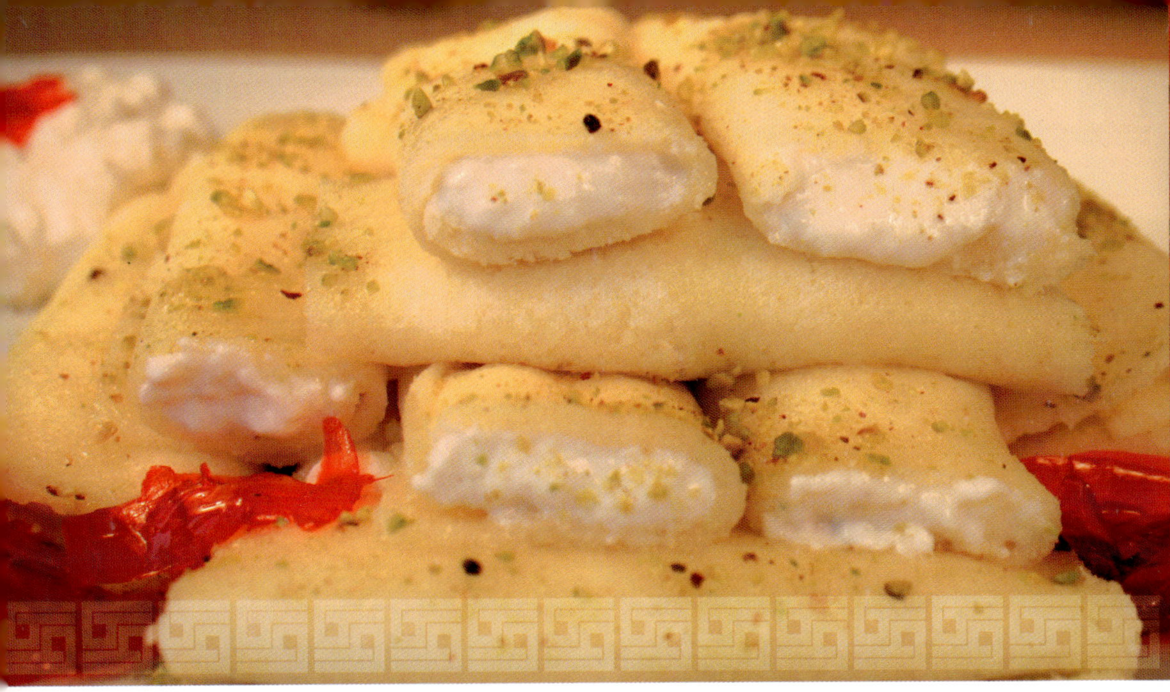

Cream-filled Cheese Fingers:
Halawet al Jiben

حلاوة الجبن

Ingredients

½ recipe Clotted Cream
1 recipe Lebanese Syrup
8 ounces fresh mozzarella cheese, unsalted
⅓ cup water
¾ cup fine farina
1 cup Lebanese Syrup
1 tablespoon orange blossom water

Rolling pin
¼ cup Lebanese Syrup
Orange flower jam (optional)
To garnish: ¼ cup crushed pistachio nuts

Start to finish
15 minutes
plus cream and
syrup recipes
Serves 8

Preparation

- Lebanese Syrup prepared and set aside
- Clotted Cream prepared and set aside

Procedure

1• Pour ⅓ cup water into a small saucepan and bring to a boil over high heat.

2• Cut cheese into thin slices, add to the boiling water and stir until cheese is melted.

3• Add ¼ cup syrup, stir and reduce heat to medium; gradually add farina while stirring quickly.

4• Pour orange blossom water over the mixture and stir until well combined. Turn off heat and transfer dough onto a large working area coated with ¼ cup syrup.

5• Roll out the dough, add the remaining syrup and continue rolling the dough until it is very thin, ⅛ inch in thickness or less.

6• Slice dough into 3 x 4 inch pieces. Place 1 tablespoon clotted cream in a thin row by one edge of each piece, then roll individually to form cheese fingers and transfer onto a platter.

7• Pour ¼ cup syrup over the rolled cheese fingers and garnish the top with leftover cream and orange flower jam. Sprinkle with crushed pistachio nuts and serve.

Serve cold or at room temperature for dessert or breakfast.

Nutrition Information per Serving

Calories 233, Fat 6g, Saturated fat 3.5g, Cholesterol 20mg, Carbohydrate 38g, Fiber 1g, Protein 7g

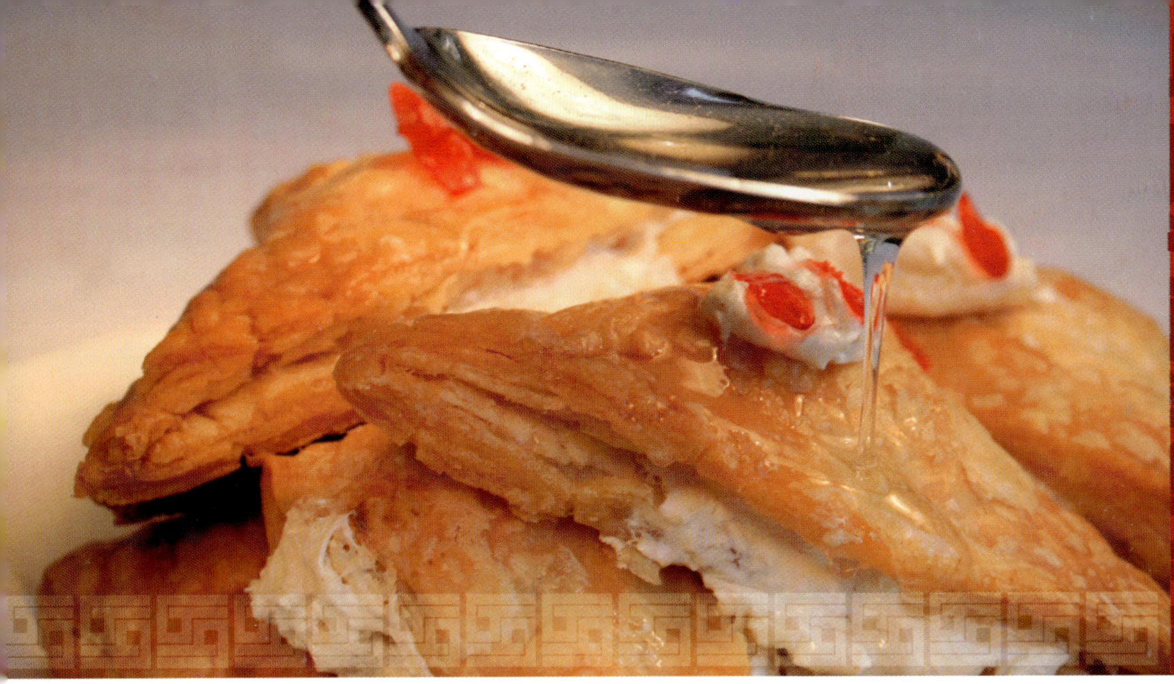

Cream-filled Puff Pastry:

Warbet bil Kashta

وربات بالقشطه

Ingredients

½ recipe Clotted Cream
½ recipe Lebanese Syrup
5 sheets of 5 x 5-inch puff pastry at room temperature

Cookie sheet
2 tablespoons melted butter
Pastry brush
To garnish: ½ cup crushed pistachio nuts

Start to finish
30 minutes
plus clotted cream
and syrup recipes
Serves 10

Preparation

- Clotted Cream recipe prepared and set aside
- Lebanese Syrup recipe prepared and set aside

Procedure

1• Preheat oven to 350 degrees F.

2• Place one sheet of puff pastry on a cutting board and cut it diagonally with a sharp knife to make 2 triangles.

3• Gently fold one triangle and press the two ends of one side together firmly to form a smaller triangle. Pick it up in your hand, place approximately 2 tablespoons of clotted cream inside and close the opening firmly.

4• Finish the other triangle in the same way and place them both on a cookie sheet ¼ inch apart. Reserve any leftover cream.

5• Follow the same steps to finish the remaining sheets. Brush the tops of the finished pastries with butter and bake them for 15 minutes, or until they are golden brown.

6• Place a baked pastry on a dessert plate and top it with a dab of leftover cream, a teaspoon of crushed pistachio nuts and syrup to your taste.

Serve hot or at room temperature with syrup for dessert.

Nutrition Information per Serving

Calories 248, Fat 11g, Saturated fat 4g, Cholesterol 18mg, Carbohydrate 35g, Fiber 1g, Protein 4g

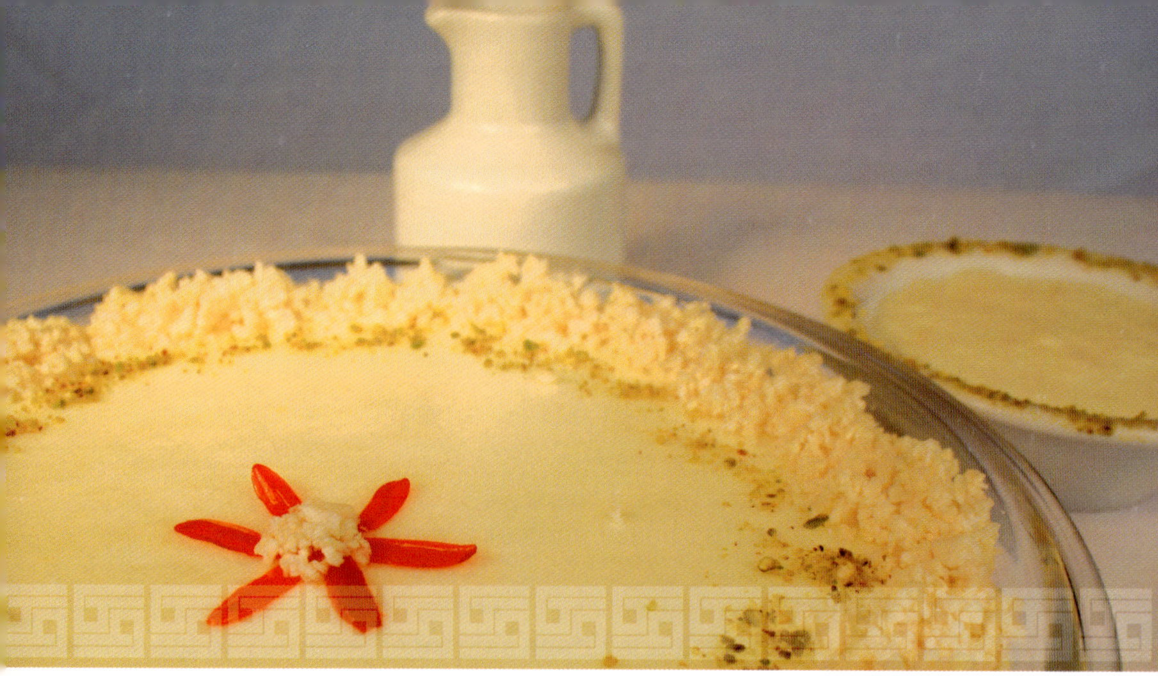

Milk Pudding: M'hallabyeh

مهلبيه

Ingredients

1 recipe Lebanese Syrup
6 cups whole milk
½ cup cornstarch
½ teaspoon sugar
⅛ teaspoon or a small head miskeh
1 tablespoon orange blossom water

Food processor
1 cup almonds
To Garnish: ¼ cup pistachio nuts

Start to Finish
20 minutes
plus syrup recipe
Serves 6

Preparation

• Lebanese Syrup recipe prepared and set aside
• Place sugar and miskeh on a flat platter, smash them with the bottom of a flat cup and set aside.
• Crush almonds and pistachio nuts separately in a food processor and set aside.

Procedure

1• Pour 5 cups of milk into a large pot. In a small bowl, combine cornstarch and milk, stir well to dissolve and pour it through a sifter into the pot.

2• Stir with a wooden spoon and place over medium-high heat. Continue to stir regularly until it boils and thickens, about 12 minutes.

3• Reduce heat to medium, stir in miskeh mixture and continue to stir while adding blossom water, then turn off heat.

4• Pour milk pudding into a large, deep platter and set aside to cool, then refrigerate.

5• Once it is cold, top pudding with crushed almonds and garnish with pistachio nuts. Serve it with the syrup.

Serve it cold for dessert.

** TIP Lebanese Syrup can be prepared a few days in advance. Milk Pudding can be prepared 5 days in advance if kept covered in the refrigerator. You can serve it with jam or honey instead of syrup. Miskeh (licorice flavored resin from the pistacia lenliscus tree) is used to flavor sweets. It must be pulverized with a mortar and pestle before using it.*

Nutrition Information per Serving

Calories 342, Fat 19g, Saturated fat 4g, Cholesterol 17mg, Carbohydrate 32g, Fiber 3g, Protein 14g

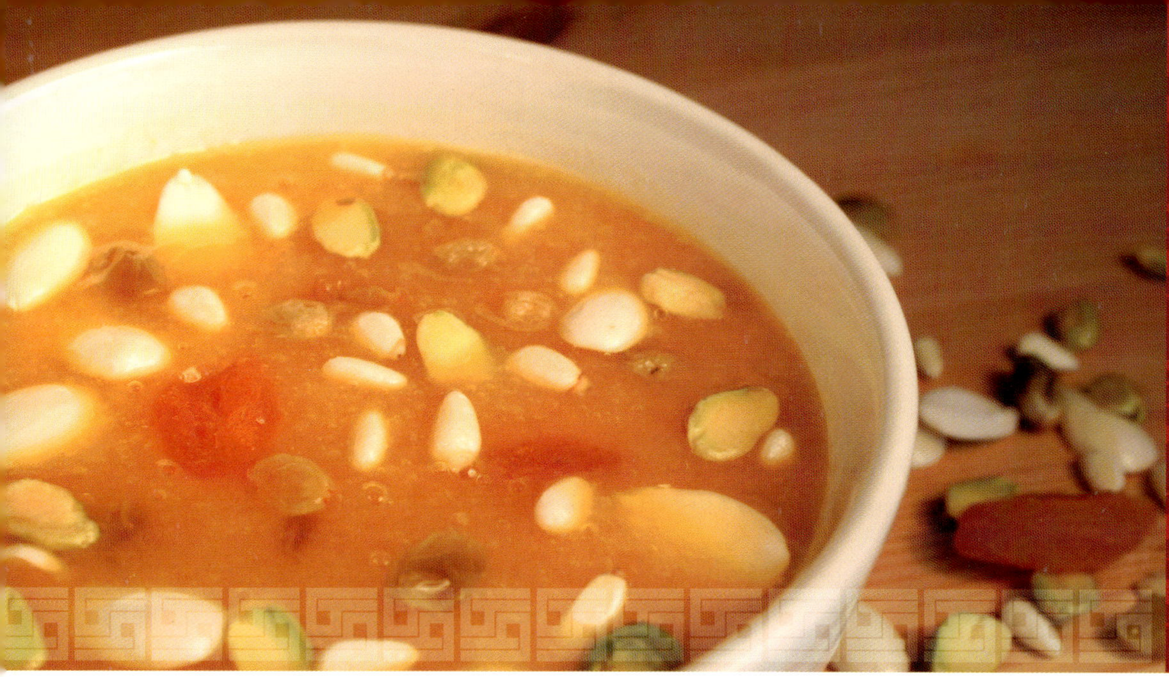

Ramadan Treat: Khoo'shaf

خوشاف

Ingredients

16 oz. dried apricot paste
6 cups water
Sugar or to taste

Electric blender
Fine sifter
½ cup blanched pistachio nuts
½ cup blanched almonds, sliced
½ cup pine nuts
½ cup dried apricots
½ cup yellow raisins

Start to Finish
10 minutes
plus soaking time
Serves 8

Preparation

- Cut dried apricot paste into little pieces and soak in 2 cups water overnight.
- Soak each type of nut separately in ½ cup water for half an hour or overnight in the refrigerator in covered containers.

Procedure

1• Place soaked apricot paste and the 2 cups water into the blender and process until well blended. Add another 4 cups of water and process thoroughly to combine.

2• Pour mixture through a fine sifter into a large bowl.

3• Drain pistachio nuts, pine nuts and almonds and add to the bowl, along with the apricots and raisins. Refrigerate for an hour and serve.

Serve it cold for dessert in the fasting month or as a year-round treat.

** TIP Ramadan Treat stays fresh up to a week if refrigerated in a covered container. Dried apricot paste is similar to the popular fruit roll-up. It comes in a 1-pound package and can be cut to the desired amount.*

Nutrition Information per Serving

Calories 332, Fat 14g, Saturated fat 1g, Cholesterol 0mg, Carbohydrate 52g, Fiber 7g, Protein 7g

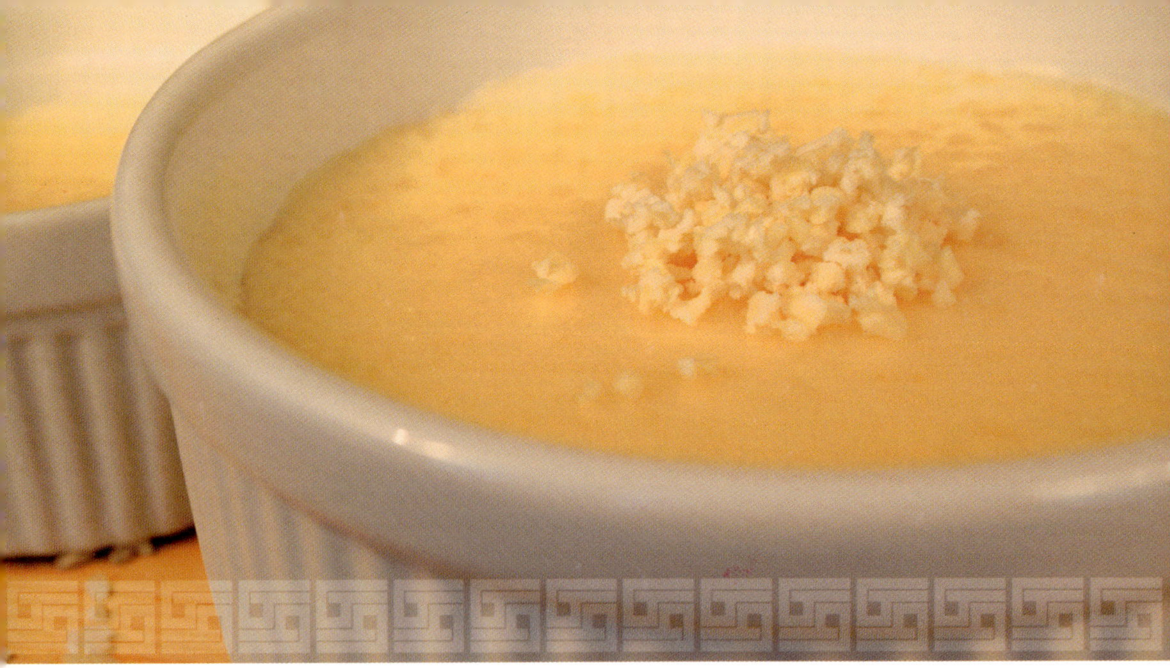

Rice Pudding: Riz b'Haleeb

رز بحليب

Ingredients

¼ cup short grain rice soaked in
⅓ cup water for 10 minutes
6 cups whole milk
⅓ cup sugar
1 tablespoon cornstarch
1 tablespoon water
1 teaspoon orange blossom water (optional)

Medium stainless steel pot
6 small bowls
¼ cup crushed, blanched almonds (optional)

Start to Finish
1 hour
Serves 6

Procedure

1• Place rice and water in the pot and soak for 10 minutes. Add milk to the rice and bring to a boil over high heat, stirring constantly. Be careful, the rice sticks easily to the bottom.

2• Reduce heat to medium and stir frequently until the rice is soft, about 20 minutes.

3• Add sugar and stir thoroughly. Reduce heat to medium-low and stir often until it thickens, about 10 more minutes.

4• Mix cornstarch with 1 tablespoon water. Add cornstarch mixture to the pot while stirring and adjust heat to medium-high. Continue to stir for 7 minutes, then blend in orange blossom water and turn off heat.

5• Transfer pudding into 6 small bowls. Once they cool, top each bowl with 1 tablespoon almonds (optional) and serve.

Serve it hot, warm or cold with or without almonds for dessert, snack or breakfast.

** TIP Rice Pudding stays fresh up to a week if kept covered in the refrigerator.*

Nutrition Information per Serving

Calories 221, Fat 5g, Saturated fat 3g, Cholesterol 17mg, Carbohydrate 37g, Fiber 0g, Protein 8g

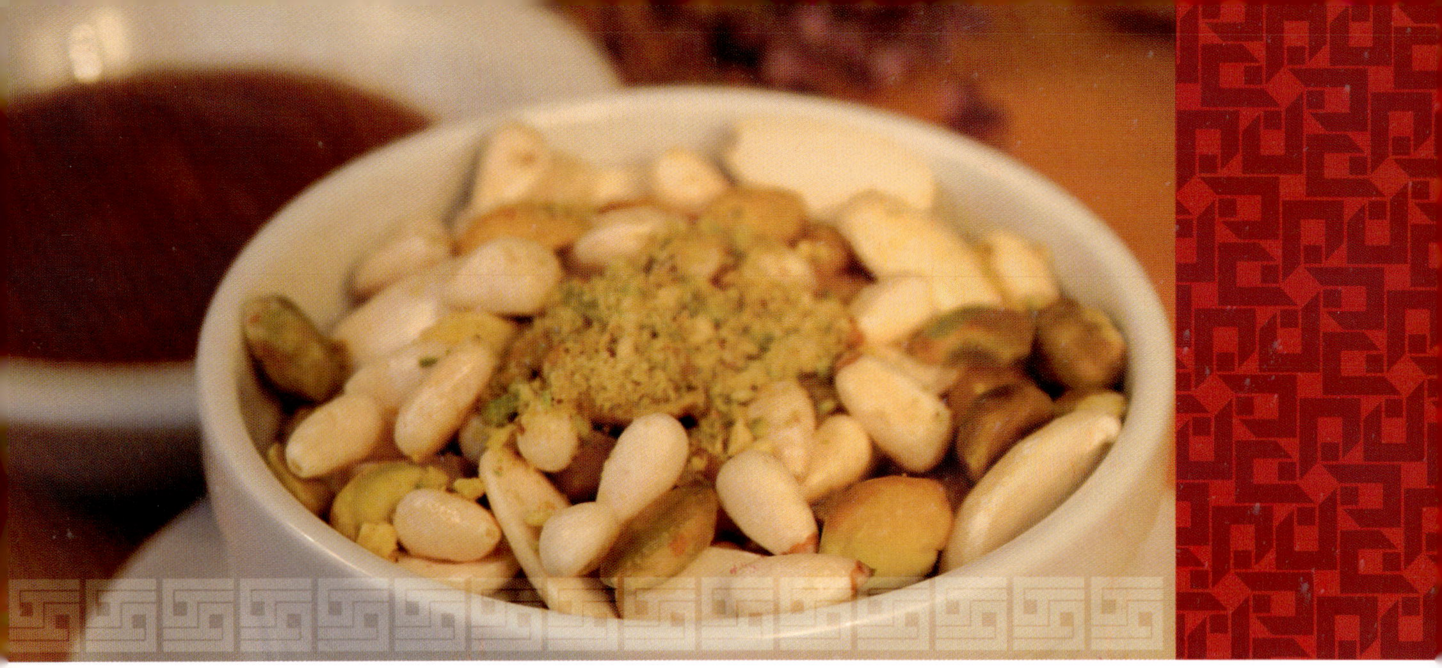

Special treat is for special occasions. It is always served when guests drop by to congratulate the new parents on the birth of their baby.

Special Treat: : Moghli

مغلي

Ingredients

1 cup rice powder
2 cups sugar
1 tablespoon ground caraway seeds
2 tablespoons ground cinnamon
6 cups water

1 cup ground coconut, unsweetened
½ cup peeled almonds, sliced
½ cup pine nuts
½ cup crushed walnuts
½ cup peeled pistachio nuts

Start to Finish
20 minutes
Serves 6

Preparation

- Soak all nuts in water in separate container for an hour or overnight.

Procedure

1• In a large pot, combine rice, sugar, caraway and cinnamon. Slowly pour in water while stirring and place over medium heat.

2• Continue to stir and bring to a boil for 5 minutes. Once mixture thickens, turn off heat and set aside.

3• With a ladle, pour mixture into small bowls and set aside to cool, and then refrigerate.

4• Serve it cold with 2 teaspoons each of coconut, almonds, pine nuts, walnuts and pistachio nuts as a topping.

Serve it hot, warm or cold with or without almonds for dessert, snack or breakfast.

**TIP Special Treat will stay fresh up to a week if kept covered in the refrigerator.*
Peeled almonds and pistachio nuts can be found at most Mediterranean or international markets.
To peel almonds cover them with water and microwave them for 2 or 3 minutes, then drain – the peels will come off easily.

Nutrition Information per Serving

Calories 573, Fat 25g, Saturated fat 2.5g, Cholesterol 0mg, Carbohydrate 85g, Fiber 4g, Protein 8g

Table of Nutrient Analysis

Appetizers	CALORIES	PROTEIN	CARBS	FIBER	FAT	SAT	MUF	PUF	CHOL	SODIUM	GOOD SOURCE
Eggplant Dip	117	4	15	5	6	1	2	2.5	0		B Vitamins
Vegetarian Patties	256	10.5	31	9.5	10.5	1	3.5	6	0		Folate
Chick-peas Puree	180	6.5	16	4	11	1.5	5	4.5	0		B Vitamins
Red Peppers	95	2	8	2	7	1	3	3	0		Vitamin A, Vitamin C
Swisschard with Peas	182	5	15	4	12	2	4	6	0		Vitamin A, Vitamin C
Fava Beans with Garlic & Tomato	691	24	65	17.5	38	11	21	4	22	935	Folate
Lebanese Couscous	414	13	71	6.5	9	4	3	1.2	14	627	Selenium, B vitamins
Pita Bread	162	6	34	2	0	0	0	0	0	223	
Cheese Tart	209	9	20	1	10	6	3	0	38	568	
Thyme Tart	129	3	19	1	5	1	3	1	0	74	
Spinach with Onions	27	1	2	1	2	0	1	0	0	25	Vitamin A, Folate, Vitamin C
Spinach Pie	151	4	21	2	6	1	4	0	0	26	Vitamin A, Folate, Vitamin C
Spinach Pie Dough	124	3	19	1	4	1	3	0	0	1	
Potato with Cilantro	184	3	29	3	7	1	2	3	0	344	Vitamin C, Vitamin B 6, Magnesium
Rice & Vegetable Pie	640	14	106	7	17	2	5	8	0	235	Selenium

Soups and Salads	CALORIES	PROTEIN	CARBS	FIBER	FAT	SAT	MUF	PUF	CHOL	SODIUM	GOOD SOURCE
Lentil Soup	413	20	54	17	14	2	10	2	0	505	Zinc, Iron, Magnesium, Vitamin B6, Folate
Lentils with Swisschard & Lemon Juice	333	18	45	16	10	1	7	2	0	519	Zinc, Iron, Magnesium, B Vitamins, Folate, Vitamin C
Mixed Grain Soup	230	10	29	8	9	1	5	2	60	217	Selenium, Zinc, Magnesium, Folate, B Vitamins
Vemicelli Soup	234	16	14	2	13	6	5	1	0	681	Selenium, Zinc, Vitamin B12
Arugula & Watercress Salad	93	1	3	0	9	1	7	1	0	8	
Cabbage Salad	140	1	5	2	14	2	10	2	0	16	Vitamin C
Chickpea & Tomato Salad	469	20	66	19	15	2	8	4	0	513	Selenium, Zinc, Iron, Folate, Vitamin C
Salad with Toasted Bread	244	5	27	4	14.5	2	10	1.5	0		Vitamin C
Fresh Oregano & Green Olives	95	0	2	0	10	1	7	1	0	289	Vitamin C
Yogurt & Cucumber	122	9.5	15.5	1	3	2	1	0	10		Calcium
Yogurt with Wheat	172	13	21	2.5	4	2	1	1	10		Calcium, B Vitamins
Tabouleh	188	3	15	4.5	14	2	10	2	0		Vitamin A, Vitamin C

Main course	CALORIES	PROTEIN	CARBS	FIBER	FAT	SAT	MUF	PUF	CHOL	SODIUM	GOOD SOURCE
Kibbeh Dough	180	12	14	3	8	3	3	1	54	317	Selenium, Zinc, B Vitamins
Baked Kibbeh	348	26	2	3	20	7	8	3	81	510	Selenium, Zinc, B Vitamins
Chick-peas with Bread and Yogurt	321	17	31	8	10	4	3	3	15		Calcium, B Vitamins
Lebanese Spaghetti	425	18	58	3	13	5	4	3	20		Calcium
Baby Okra with Tomato & Garlic	373	11	43	11	20	2	10	11	0	427	
Green Beans	120	1	7	3	10	1	7	1	0	5	
Mousakaa	199	7	32	11	6	1	2	3	0	113	Selenium, Zinc, Magnesium, Calcium, Folate, Vitamin C
Cracke Wheat with Chick-peas	451	18	69	18	14	2	8	3	0	573	Iron, Magnesium, B Vitamins
Cracked Wheat with Lentils	429	20	52	19	17	2	12	2	0	584	Iron, Zinc, B Vitamins
Rice with Lentils	503	17	83	11	11	1	8	1	0	315	Iron, Magnesium, Folate
Rice with Vermicelli	314	5	61	0	5	1	2	2	0	6	
Green Bean Stew	241	15	6	2	17	8	6	1	70	268	Selenium, Zinc, Vitamin B12, Niacin
Lamb Stew with Baby Okra	284	16	9	3	21	7	8	4	59	614	Selenium, Zinc, B Vitamins
Navy Bean & Lamb Stew	389	25	34	9	17	8	6	1	67	960	Selenium, Zinc, Iron, Magnesium, B Vitamins
Pea Stew with Cilantro	234	15	17	5	13	6	4	1	53	888	Zinc, Niacin, Thiamin, Vitamin A

Spinach Stew	330	29	10	6	21	6	8	4	75	534	Vitamin A
Vegetarian Grape Leaves	359	10	59	7	11	1	7	2	0	877	Selenium, Zinc, Iron, Magnesium, Calcium, B Vitamins, Vitamin C
Vegetarian Stuffed Squash	386	8	59	5	14	2	10	2	0	359	Magnesium, Vitamin C, B Vitamins
Kafta in Pita Bread	407	27	34	2	17	5.5	7	2.5	75	635	Selenium, Zinc, Vitamin B12
Leg of Lamb	387	30	6	1	26	11	11	2.5	115	490	Selenium, Zinc, Vitamin B12, Niacin
Top Sirloin Beef	423	42	3.5	0	29	9	10.5	2.5	125	578	Selenium, Zinc, Vitamin B12, Vitamin B6, Niacin
Chicken Broth	172	26	1	0	7	2	2	1.5	79	371	Selenium, Zinc, B Vitamins
Chicken with Lemon & Garlic	399	41	15	1	18.5	4	6	6	123	732	Selenium, Zinc, B Vitamins
Chicken with Molokhia	158	17	4	1	8	3.5	2.5	1	59	277	Selenium, Zinc, B Vitamins
Chicken with Rice, Meat &Nuts	805	52	66	3	36	8	14	11	139	627	Selenium, Zinc, Iron, Magnesium, B Vitamins
Baked Fish Filets in Garlic Sauce	275	32	1	0	15	2	11	1	44	138	Selenium, B Vitamins
Fish with Rice & Nuts	534	30	44	3	27	2.5	10	12	29	93	Selenium, Zinc, Iron, Magnesium, B Vitamins, Vitamin E
Shrimp with Cilantro & Garlic	249	23	4	1	15	2	10	2	166	500	Selenium
Tahini Sauce with Pine Nuts	128	3	4	1	12	1	5	5	0	15	

On the Grill	CALORIES	PROTEIN	CARBS	FIBER	FAT	SAT	MUF	PUF	CHOL	SODIUM	GOOD SOURCE
Chicken Kebabs	403	45	13	3	18	4	9	3	122	586	Selenium, Vitamin C
Kafta Kebabs	292	29	3	0	17	7	8	1	100	445	Selenium, Zinc, B Vitamins
Lamb Kebabs	406	29	10	2	27	11	13	2	109	453	Selenium, Zinc, B Vitamins
Liver Kebabs	175	22	4	0	8	2	2	2	358	335	Selenium, Zinc, Iron, B Vitamins, Vitamin A
Shrimp Kebabs	138	12	1	0	9	2	6	1	88	246	Selenium
Grilled Chicken	412	42	1	0	25	6	11	5	137	634	Selenium
Grilled Eggplant	132	2	13	7	9	1	7	1	0	5	Vitamin C
Whole Grilled Trout	187	20	1	0	11	2	5	3	56	300	Selenium, B Vitamins

Dessert	CALORIES	PROTEIN	CARBS	FIBER	FAT	SAT	MUF	PUF	CHOL	SODIUM	GOOD SOURCE
Baklava	334	5	29	2	22	9	8	4	35	252	
Lebanese Syrup	81	0	21	0	0	0	0	0	0	12	
Clotted Cream	95	2	9	0	6	3.5	2	0	18	91	Calcium
Cream-Filled Cheese Fingers	233	7	38	1	6	3.5	2	0	20	175	Calcium
Cream-filled Puff Pastry	248	4	35	1	11	4	4	2	18	105	
Bird Nest with Pistachio	107	2	15	1	5	1	2	1	3	12	
Holiday Pastry Dough	60	1	9	0	2	1	1	0	5	16	Selenium, B Vitamins
Pistachio-Filled Pastry	115	3	14	1	5	2	2	1	5	17	B Vitamins
Walnut-Filled Pastry	123	2	14	1	7	2	1	3	5	16	Selenium, B Vitamins
Easter Biscuits	79	1	17	0	1	1	0	0	1	5	
Ramadan Treat	332	7	52	7	14	1	6	5	0	8	Magnesium, Vitamin A, Vitamin E
Special Treat	573	8	85	4	25	2.5	9	11	0	71	Vitamin E
Cream of Wheat Cake	278	4	49	1	8	3	3	1	14	57	B Vitamins
Rice Pudding	221	8	37	0	5	3	1	0	17	100	Calcium
Milk Pudding	342	14	32	3	19	4	10	4	17	117	

www.aldoukan.com
www.lebanesefoodmarket.com

Caravan Foods
Mideastern/European
2817 N. Country Club Road
Tucson AZ 85716
(520)323-6808

Baiz Market
523 N 20th St
Phoenix, AZ 85006
(602) 252-8996

Middle Eastern Bakery Deli
3052 N 16TH St
Phoenix, AZ 85016
(602) 277-4927
spicebazaar.com

17th Street Market
830 E. 17th Street
Tucson, AZ 85719
(520) 884-9554

نارة porfavor
Dam W Fares, Achir Dayeh Str.
Tripoli Lebanon
Tel: 06 - 411410

Index:

Safa Merheb was born and raised in Tripoli, north of Beirut, Lebanon. As a young child, she enjoyed observing her mother prepare the daily, mid-day meal, and sometimes her tiny hands helped to stir the rice pudding or roll the grape leaves

When she married and left her homeland for Tucson, Arizona, she faced the challenge of preparing these same Lebanese dishes for her family thousands of miles from home, with recipes that had been handed down verbally from mother to daughter. Safa also experienced the time crunch of the busy American woman as she raised three children and worked as an early childhood educator.

She succeeded in providing her family with traditional, home-cooked Mediterranean cuisine with a combination of determination, good planning and the use of cooking techniques detailed in her book. She even found time to teach Lebanese cooking classes in her community and to consult for a Mediterranean restaurant. The inspiration for writing this book came from her family and friends, who appreciated her authentic dishes and encouraged her to pass them to the next generation in a quick and easy-to-use form.

The result, "The Pure Taste of Lebanon from Safa's Kitchen," contains recipes that are adapted to employ modern tools to make them easy, simple and quick, and still ensure that the traditional flavor of the Lebanese cuisine is preserved.

The Pure Taste of Lebanon from Safa's Kitchen:

• Is a book that captures the pure taste of Lebanon, and enables everyday people to recreate it,

• Introduces easy cooking tips that motivate family and kids to gather and cook together,

• Has more than 70 Authentic recipes divided into 5 categories, with tips to guide you when and what to serve it with,

• Includes nutritional information per serving for the calorie counters of the world,

• Teaches specific strategies and techniques for preparing an easy, fresh, and healthy gourmet meal in no time for our busy daily lives,

• Instructions are giving in the clearest and most accessible way for the modern cook who enjoy Lebanese cuisine and who seek to try new ethnic recipes.

Often cooks are deterred from trying new recipes that include new flavors due to the unavailability of ingredients. Most of these recipes use ingredients readily available in local supermarkets. For those "hard-to-find" ingredients in the more exotic recipes, "The Pure Taste of Lebanon from Safa's Kitchen" supplies Internet addresses that provide online ordering and local Middle Eastern grocery stores.